The
Stork Club

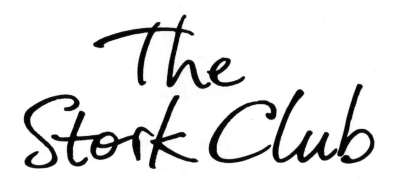

The Stork Club

One woman's journey to the front
line of fertility

IMOGEN EDWARDS-JONES

BANTAM PRESS

LONDON • TORONTO • SYDNEY • AUCKLAND • JOHANNESBURG

TRANSWORLD PUBLISHERS
61–63 Uxbridge Road, London W5 5SA
a division of The Random House Group Ltd

RANDOM HOUSE AUSTRALIA (PTY) LTD
20 Alfred Street, Milsons Point, Sydney,
New South Wales 2061, Australia

RANDOM HOUSE NEW ZEALAND LTD
18 Poland Road, Glenfield, Auckland 10, New Zealand

RANDOM HOUSE SOUTH AFRICA (PTY) LTD
Isle of Houghton, Corner of Boundary and Carse O'Gowrie Roads,
Houghton 2198, South Africa

Published 2006 by Bantam Press
a division of Transworld Publishers

A catalogue record for this book is available from the British Library.
ISBN 9780593056080 (from Jan 07)
ISBN 0593056086

Typeset in 11/18pt Goudy by
Falcon Oast Graphic Art Ltd

Printed in Great Britain by
Clays Ltd, Bungay, Suffolk

1 3 5 7 9 10 8 6 4 2

Papers used by Transworld Publishers are natural, recyclable products
made from wood grown in sustainable forests. The manufacturing
processes conform to the environmental regulations of the
country of origin.

For Less Attractive, who made everything better,
and Miss Milk, who made it all worth while

But once in a while the odd thing happens
Once in a while the dream comes true
And the whole pattern of life is altered
Once in a while the moon turns blue

W. H. Auden

Introduction

It was a long time before I realized I had a problem. It sort of crept up on me and took me over without me really noticing. One minute I was a normal woman, going about her business, thinking that it was time to get around to having a baby, and the next, I was this needy mad thing sticking needles into my feet, drinking pomegranate juice, chasing my husband round the room demanding sex. This vague desire to have a baby, a dull, niggling ache, had almost overnight mutated into an over-powering, all-encompassing hunger that caught me by surprise.

And I'm not normally a hormonal type of person. I like to think that I am quite rational, quite focused. I'm of the school of thought that if you want something all you have to do is concentrate and work hard enough, and with dedication, determination and a little luck, you can usually manage it. However, in the baby stakes this was clearly not the case, for no amount of concentration, or willpower, or indeed sex, was getting me pregnant.

I kept quiet about it at first. Well, no one wants to look like a failure, particularly when everyone around them seems to be managing it all so easily. In a society where success is instant and no one saves or waits for anything any more, I didn't want to be the only person who couldn't achieve. When everyone else is having it all, it doesn't do to be the one person not capable of doing the basics. I was bad at being female, and that's not something anyone wants to talk about.

Then, after about a year of silence, I couldn't take the secrecy any more. I had begun to avoid girlfriends who were pregnant and to greet each joyous conception with an increasingly sour demeanour. Not that I wished any of them any ill, it was just a bit too painful to have one's barrenness reflected back at one all the time. So I started to talk about it. Drunkenly at first, weeping into my wine at three in the morning, I'd grab some poor unsuspecting girlfriend and share my predicament (or lack of it). I'd tell them that we had been trying for ages. I'd say that the baby sex was becoming a nightmare and that we were thinking about other ways that were less to do with what nature intended and more to do with science. More often than not, they would open up too. Nearly all of them had either had a similar experience or had heard a similar story from a friend of theirs.

There seemed to be this great conspiracy of silence. One in six couples have trouble conceiving and no one ever really talks about it. Women all over the UK are having all sorts of fertility treatment, including IVF, and they are doing it on the quiet. This suddenly struck me as ridiculous and extremely unhelpful. Why, when you are at your most vulnerable and low, are you not allowed to talk about it? Why should you have to smile stiffly through your Sunday lunch as, yet again, some aged aunt tactlessly asks you why you don't have children? Why should you be seen as a failure for finding it difficult to conceive? Why are we all so worried about what other people think? Why are we all so embarrassed to be seen to try and fail?

So instead of suffering in silence, hiding that fact that my life wasn't going to plan, I decided I'd write about it all: the highs, the lows, the tears, the hell, the nightmare, the misery, the sadness and eventually the overwhelming joy in a column,

Shall I be a mother?, in the pages of the *Daily Telegraph*.

Every other week for nearly two years, for better or for worse, I shared my IVF story. And the feedback I had from these columns was extraordinary. I had letters from elderly majors whose wives had had problems in the Fifties. I had letters from mothers whose daughters were doing IVF, from young women in the same situation as I, and I had card after card from husbands whose wives were miserable and high on hormones and who were finding it difficult to talk. During the months I wrote the column I struck up penpal friendships with lots of readers. Some sent me good luck charms, others presents, but mostly I received treatment updates with terribly sad news and occasionally delightful joy. These columns were, possibly, the way I kept sane – although some would beg to differ. They were, however, certainly the way I found out that I was not alone in my agony and pain. I found them useful and I hope that if you or someone you know is about to go down the rocky road of fertility treatment, you will too.

It is a long and fraught journey that is full of great lows and potentially great highs, where no matter how miserable and isolated you feel, it is important to try to remember who you are and – if at all possible – to retain a sense of humour.

So here is my story.

1

When I was a teenager I thought you could get pregnant sitting in a jacuzzi. I'm not sure I even knew what a jacuzzi was, but I knew they were racy places where racy things happened. Men, as far as I remember, didn't even have to be there. Just so long as they'd been in the water in some sort of excitable state, then pregnancy was inevitable – even if you kept your pants on. You see, pregnancy was that easy, that dangerous, and it could ruin your life.

Almost twenty years later and pregnancy may still ruin my life – although this time it is not the threat of what having a baby would do (no school, no education, no career, no future) but of not having a baby at all. I have been trying to get pregnant for two years and not even come close to the pitter-patter of tiny feet.

Looking back now at my libidinous twenties, all the signs of my current childlessness were there: I just failed to notice them. For all my fooling around, I never once had a close shave or scare. I've lost count of how many nights I spent counselling weeping girlfriends over wine and pregnancy-testing kits. The more we drank, the more plastic sticks we'd line up, waiting, cross-eyed, for blue lines to appear. But weirdly it never happened to me. It was right at the height of AIDS awareness and we were all having sex in wetsuits, so I wasn't that surprised. And, of course, I'm quite grown up about these things. Except, actually, I'm not.

When I first hooked up with my less attractive half over ten years ago, we paid lip service to contraception, then after a while we both decided to embrace our non-existent inner Catholic selves and rely on withdrawal. This seemed to work. Seven years later we skipped un-shotgun-like down the aisle and decided that we should get cracking in earnest.

Except there is nothing more unattractive than earnest sex. And considering ourselves too groovy to be seen to try too hard, we launched into a few half-baked attempts to conceive.

We tried drunken sex, very drunken sex and occasionally hungover sex but none of it seemed to work. After about a year of pretending not to care, the tension was beginning to mount. Why wasn't this happening to us? My girlfriends were 'falling pregnant' all over the place and I was growing to hate the expression, as if accidentally tumbling over something could spontaneously get you up the duff. But for some of them it was true. 'It wasn't really planned,' they'd giggle into their Starbucks. 'You know, it was just one of those drunken weekends.' Oh good, I'd smile, lucky old you.

It was probably time to get myself checked out. One of my great friends suggested a handsome gynaecologist, Mr Henderson, who works out of a baronial hall in Harley Street. He'd seen more glamorous bits than a Manhattan fannicurist, she warned me, so he was definitely a best-pants kind of doctor. I walked into his suite sporting my one pair of La Perla. He was foolishly nice to me and I promptly burst into tears. Perhaps this baby thing was getting to me more than I'd thought? He gave my womb the onceover and pronounced that it was working well and, in fact, if I looked closely I'd see that I was ovulating right now and should go home and have sex tonight.

'What, tonight?' I gulped.

He nodded. 'It would be a good idea.' Five hours later Less Attractive and I were flailing around like two slowly asphyxiating plaice, desperately trying to 'make a baby'. It was as sexy as a lard sandwich and still, somewhat shockingly for us both, I didn't get pregnant.

It was at this stage that some of my less sensitive girlfriends started to throw their helpful little oars in. One suggested that perhaps if I was really serious about babies I should cut out 'all that alcohol you drink'. Another kindly brought round a pamphlet entitled something like 'Managing Your Infertility'. And another opined, while shoving her big blue-veined breast in her newborn's mouth, that perhaps I wasn't 'psychologically ready' for children and didn't actually want them, 'otherwise you would have had one by now'.

Things were clearly getting competitive. Why wasn't I able to do what everyone else seemed to be pulling off at the weekend? Less Attractive rather bravely went to have his sperm tested and was thrilled to announce to the world that he was 'all man and had sperm like whitebait'. So it was down to me. Back to Henderson I went, and we started a course of ovarian follicle tracking. This basically meant that, with the aid of a long condom-clad probe, he could tell me exactly when I was ovulating and exactly when Less Attractive and I should get cracking.

And so the misery of 'baby sex' began in earnest. Standing at home on a Tuesday night, racy knickers at the ready, trying to initiate another spontaneous procreative session, was exhausting and no fun at all. The evenings when we were supposed to be 'doing it' were a nightmare. We would get tense and bicker. I turned into some hideous moaning sex-demanding harridan and he'd get all huffy, annoyed and 'tired'. We'd have whole weekends of it. I'd dress up like Britney Spears and sit there like a tethered goat waiting for him to feel he was up to the job. It was like something out of a really lame porn film. Then one night he came home and announced he had a new plan, and he was just going to 'surprise' me with it. I have to say that being bent double on the sofa, suffocating on my fun-fur cushion while listening to Sharon row on *EastEnders* is not my idea of a good surprise. But, you know, each to their own.

We were still getting nowhere. Perhaps it was time to see if there was something seriously wrong. Henderson suggested a hysterosalpingogram. This is surely a procedure invented by a man. I wish blokes had to consent to someone pushing a blunt instrument right up through their bits and then releasing a whole load of dye down the appropriate tubes while they were X-rayed for blockages or the odd impasse. In short, it was agony. In fact, the only good news to come from all that unpleasantness was that my tubes (the width of a human hair) were clear, open and ready to go.

Just to get things moving along nicely, Henderson suggested a short course of the fertility pill Clomid, which he described as his favourite drug. Now I've had my fair share of supposedly 'amusing' drugs, but none quite so relentlessly unpleasant as Clomid. There were tears, painful breasts, tantrums, and an inner anger that would never go away. I also began to pile on weight like I was already pregnant. I felt too fat for sex. They also made both Less Attractive and me paranoid that it was only a matter of a quick one before we'd be on the phone to Max Clifford announcing our terrifying multi-birth to the world.

But the Clomid seemed to make no difference. Then, after about six months, something happened. I was fat and foul-tempered, which was not unusual; however, this time my period was actually late. A whole week late. I was excited. He was thrilled. I did a test, sitting in a freezing loo at six in the morning, and waited for the stick to turn blue. It didn't. I couldn't believe it. Why not? What had I done to the world to make it not happen? I'm afraid I went out that night and got more plastered than is dignified. I think 'absolutely ratted' is the expression.

Anyway, three days later I had a miscarriage. It came as a bit of a shock. Turned out I had been pregnant after all. They are not pleasant things, miscarriages, but for some reason best known to myself I decided that the show must go on regardless. I vaguely remember sitting in a girlfriend's house in silent agony while she told me yet again how marvellous her new baby was, and I could only sip wine, nod and feel very sorry for myself.

Yet somehow Henderson managed to put a positive spin on things. 'You've got pregnant!' he exclaimed. 'That is such good news. You know you can do it!' It was apparently cause for celebration. In fact, it was such good news he felt that we should try artificial insemination straight away. 'Think of it like the D-day landings,' he said. 'Except instead of the sperm having to make the crossing by boat, they are choppered in, raring to go.'

Well, it was more than the sperm that was raring to go. Two days before schedule I ovulated and suddenly had to get Less Attractive out of some VIP meeting. He rushed home mid-morning to provide his deposit. Careering down the stairs with his trousers round his ankles, he handed over a rather empty-looking pot.

'That it?' I said.

11

'Sorry,' he replied. 'I kind of missed.'

But there was no turning back. I drove like a maniac across town, my husband's sperm sample snug between my breasts – on doctor's orders, I assure you. The sperm was then put through various gymnastic running and jumping tests, which amazingly it passed, and I was left with a pink phial of washed and manicured superseed.

Insemination was like all the other gynaecological treatments before it. They said it wouldn't hurt at all, it hurt quite a lot and then you forget about it and think only of the results. There followed a tense no-drinking, no-smoking, no-fun two weeks while we waited, quietly confident this time. It must have worked. After all, how lazy can sperm be? They'd been delivered to the point of contact, what more did they want?

Well, apparently a whole lot more than a free ride. It failed. So we tried again and it failed again. And now I have been recommended IVF. I have to say I'm feeling deeply apprehensive. If I'm honest, I'm really not sure how much more of this I can take. With all the highs, the lows, the weight gain, the mood swings, the depression and the very great upset every time it doesn't work, I am feeling exhausted. But I can't not go for it. I am thirty-six years old. I have what is known as 'unexplained infertility', and nearly £5,000 worth of IVF is my only option left.

There are some people who moan about IVF, saying that it is not a woman's 'right' to have a child. However, suddenly finding myself in this position, the question of right simply doesn't occur to me. It's more like by any means necessary. The fertility game is like one long marathon where you just have to keep on running. No matter how many times the finish line is moved, no matter how increasingly hard the road or unpleasant the terrain, you pick yourself up and ever more determinedly you keep on going. Until one day you hope, you pray, you just might make it.

2

So here I am at the Assisted Conception Unit of the Lister Hospital. In a red-brick piece of modernized Victoriana just off Chelsea Bridge, it is one of those clinical, efficient places that private medicine tries to make more palatable with thick carpets, cut flowers, upmarket magazines and co-ordinated soft furnishings. The staff are welcoming and pleasant but there is no getting away from the fact that sitting here, waiting for my first IVF appointment, it is hard not to think of myself as a loser. Of all the places, in all the rooms, in all the world, I never imagined I'd end up here – perched on the edge of a well-padded chair, staring at a water cooler, trying not to catch anyone else's eye.

And to make matters worse, Less Attractive is sitting here with me, loudly reading his newspaper, texting important work people and making full use of the coffee- and tea-making facilities. This is the first time he's ventured to the fertility front line and, though he's exuding a sort of hectic confidence, there is no telling how he's going to react. All the other procedures – the artificial inseminations, the follicle tracking, the blue dye blasted up my fallopian tubes – I've been through on my own. But my husband thinks he's a modern, caring, sharing metrosexual so it will be interesting to see his limit.

No sooner do we walk into our consultant Dr Jaya Parikh's airy office than he appears to reach it. Lying on the desk, right in front of his chair, is a large black-and-white diagram of a vagina and he simply doesn't know where to look. While Dr Parikh goes through a questionnaire of both our intimate sexual histories, Less Attractive fidgets, fiddles and then with one swift hand movement, disguised by a cough, he turns the diagram over. Finally, he can concentrate.

Dr Parikh starts typing things into her computer. 'With someone as young as you, the chances of success with IVF are greatly increased,' she announces. It's the first piece of good news I've heard in two years.

'What?' I say. 'I'm young?'

Dr Parikh nods. 'Oh yes, thirty-six is young in IVF terms.'

I thought she was rather pretty when I walked into the room, but now I obviously love her. She continues typing into some special Lister Hospital computer programme that takes into account all our various health factors and then announces that I have a 52 per cent chance of getting pregnant. Bearing in mind that for a fertile woman having plenty of sex, the likelihood of getting pregnant is only about 10 per cent per cycle, this seems delightfully high. Less Attractive and I are excited.

'Your odds are good,' she says encouragingly. 'Very good.'

Dr Parikh reclaims her diagram and starts to explain the ins, outs and wherefores of IVF. Less Attractive and I stare at the large drawing. I didn't even do biology at school so am somewhat confused by the whole thing. He, on the other hand, looks like he's getting a headache.

'What? So are those fallopian tubes?' he asks, prodding away.

Dr Parikh nods.

'And where do they go?'

She shows him on the diagram.

He leans forward. 'So what's that?'

'The uterus.'

'Yuk,' he declares, sitting straight back. 'I'm glad I'm not a lady.'

Dr Parikh laughs. 'First things first,' she says. 'We put you on the pill.'

The pill? The female contraceptive pill? I'm not sure why but I start to sob. It comes from the very depths of my stomach and I can't stop it. The idea that after two years of trying to have a baby I might want to take a contraceptive is too much to deal with. It is such a directional volte-face, I can't understand it. Dr Parikh brings out her well-worn box of tissues and tries to explain the reasons behind such an apparent contradiction. It's a way of giving the ovaries a rest before the hormonal onslaught that is IVF. It is also a way of timing things correctly and taking control of your hormones. I reluctantly agree.

She then goes on to explain the rest of the process. After a month on the pill you start to sniff a drug (Synarel) that causes you to hormonally flatline and effectively puts you through the menopause. Then you inject yourself with Gonal F, which fills you full of female hormones and stimulates your follicles into producing anything up to twenty eggs, which they then harvest.

'This is when you come in,' she says, turning to Less Attractive, who shifts importantly in his seat.

'Oh yes, terribly difficult,' I say sarcastically, staring at the vagina.

'But it is,' insists Dr Parikh. 'Some men find it very stressful when it comes to giving their sample.'

Less Attractive nods with earnest interest.

'But we do provide you with magazines,' she says helpfully. 'Unlike the Chelsea and Westminster, where they actually have proper films.'

'What?' says Less Attractive, perking up no end. This is, after all, his sort of subject. 'They've got proper porn movies at the Chelsea and Westminster?'

'Oh yes,' nods Dr Parikh. 'In wide screen. On a plasma TV.'

'Darling,' he says, turning to me, his eyes wide open with concern. 'I really think we should go there.'

Ten minutes later, with stories of fertilization, implantation and success ringing in our ears, we walk out with a prescription a yard long. The list of drugs is endless but our mood has lifted. Our baby problem is now somebody else's baby problem too and it feels good to share. That's one hurdle down and only another five hundred to go.

3

Having signed on the dotted line for IVF treatment and alerted my husband's finances to prepare for sudden haemorrhaging, I decide that preparing the rest of my body for the hormonal roller coaster might also be a good idea. After all, if you are going to spend so much and put yourself through so much, you may as well optimize the likelihood of a positive outcome.

So I book myself an appointment with naturopath Max Tomlinson at Pure Medicine in Harley Street. A ridiculously good-humoured Australian in rude health, he is a bright-eyed, bushy-tailed walking advert for his own medicine. He takes a look at my eyes, my tongue, my skin and my hair and announces that the liver is the powerhouse of the body and mine, having spent nearly twenty years in happy hour, is not really in a baby-producing state. So he recommends a total liver detox, which involves no wheat, no dairy, no sugar, no alcohol, and presumably no fun at all ever again. Pizzas are out. Pasta is out. Bars of chocolate can't be glanced at for fear of contamination. Ice cream is a mere memory and even cups of coffee have to make way for tight-lipped mugs of hot water and lemon. It is a hard regime and, he warns, I might feel a whole lot worse before I feel any better.

Three days into the detox and I realize that joking is not on Max's agenda. I feel dreadful. I have a headache that is squeezing the whole right side of my head in a vice and making my right eye twitch in pain. My tongue feels like a small shagpile rug and all I want to do is sleep. Fortunately, as part of my treatment Max has also recommended a course of acupuncture. He says that a couple of sessions with Justine Hankin will go a long way towards cleansing my liver and helping me down the inhospitable IVF path. And he is not wrong. My first session with Justine is bliss. Trained in China, with a sure hand and sharp needles, she is a calm person with a mellifluous voice. She has a long history of helping women with fertility problems and nothing seems to faze her, least of all my spontaneous tears as soon as she enquires after my health. Why is it that as soon as anyone is nice to me I feel the need to cry? It is so goddam embarrassing.

She lies me down, shoves some needles in my feet, knees and hands and sorts out the headache, the fat-tongue feeling and helps the liver on its way. There are a few studies that suggest acupuncture can 'dramatically increase' the IVF success rate, but even as part of the process, as someone to talk to and someone to help regulate the impending huge hormonal swings, I can see that Justine and her needles are going to be invaluable. Poor woman, I doubt she knows what is about to hit. Then again, maybe she does. She must be used to desperate women losing their brave faces as soon as they cross her threshold.

Meanwhile, the second appointment at the Assisted Conception Unit at the Lister Hospital is all about blood. And lots of it. They take something like ten phials of the stuff. I feel like the hors d'oeuvres at a vampires' tea party. They want to test me for everything from hormone levels to sticky blood, to rubella, to something-NK cells or natural killer cells, before they can get going. The rubella thing is apparently so vital that if it turns out I managed to skip school the day they were handing out German measles (quite possible) then there would be a three-month delay to my starting IVF, while they vaccinate me and wait for my immunity to come up to speed. I call my mum to see if she can remember me having it.

'If it's the sort of jab that ruins upper arms for sleeveless dresses then I think I refused,' she informs me.

Fingers crossed it is not.

The next day, thankfully it appears that rubella is not an injection that scars the upper arms and I am indeed immune, but before we all collapse with relief I do, however, have a raised Natural Killer cell count.

'Oh,' I say, thinking it sounds very Quentin Tarantino. 'Is that serious?'

'There is an increased risk of miscarriage and reduced implantation rate,' explains the nurse.

'Right,' I say.

'Basically it means that your body identifies any sperm or embryo as the enemy and gets rid of it,' she continues. 'Your killer cells kill everything off.'

The Lister was one of the first hospitals in the country to do this NK cell test as a matter of course. Normally I would have had to go through a couple of failed IVF cycles before they would suspect anything unusual. So, in a way, I'm lucky to have found out so soon. I telephone Less Attractive and explain that I have an inner bitch that's prepared to do battle with anything, whatever the cost.

'I always knew you were poisonous,' he exclaims. 'It sort of explains everything.'

Raised NK cells don't explain everything, but they sure as hell go a step towards explaining one thing – why I haven't been getting pregnant. And the relief is amazing. Having spent two years trying to have a baby, it is an incredible feeling to know now that it is not my fault. The yoga lessons I missed. The cups of coffee I drank. The blue cheese I ate. The glasses of wine I quaffed. The cigarettes I smoked. None of these were contributing factors. It was all beyond my control. There is something technically wrong with me and I'm not in that medically unsound 'unexplained fertility' boat any more. And it feels great. Two years of tension seep away.

The other wonderful thing about having NK cells is that they can be cured. I might have to take steroids for the first three months of pregnancy. I might end up with a great big fat moon-face. I might also grow a moustache and take an unhealthy interest in javelin-throwing but, at least, there might actually be a way of getting me pregnant. I have an hour-long session of acupuncture with Justine to celebrate.

4

I spend the next month on the pill, eating nothing but fruit, vegetables and grilled fish and having a weekly session with Justine, who, I have since learned, is one of the top ten acupuncturists in the country. The result, I have to say, is quite dramatic. I've lost over a stone, my humour is erring on the pleasant, and I feel ready to face all the horrors that the IVF drugs care to throw at me.

First up is Synarel or nafarelin acetate. It comes in a small, squat bottle and is snorted like a Vick's nasal spray. It looks harmless enough. All I have to do is inhale twice a day, up each nostril, at twelve-hourly intervals. It sounds simple but it is actually quite tricky to do. How much is a snort exactly? How deeply do I have to inhale? Does it matter if I am a couple of hours late? And not only does the stuff dribble out of my nose but, when I do manage to get it in, it tastes acrid and disgusting as it trickles down the back of my throat.

Turns out that Synarel may look like a harmless cutie in a small bottle but it certainly packs a punch. I was warned I might feel a little ropy. Well, I'm afraid ropy doesn't even come close. All I can say is that I have seen my fiftysomething future and I'm terrifying. If I were Less Attractive I'd probably take a very long, very complicated one-way sailing trip as soon as I come anywhere near Changing. He's got an awful lot of tension and terse tetchiness to look forward to.

Three days into taking Synarel and I get the sort of chemical headache usually born from a crack-of-dawn night on the tiles. It sits behind my eyes and stops me from being able to think. All day, every day I feel like I have smoked thirty packets of cigarettes and knocked back a case of vodka. It is hell and makes concentrating on anything a nightmare. I also have the temper of a witch. I have developed a sort of general malaise and a boiling inner anger that needs only the slightest inconvenience for it to bubble over. I shout at my sister. I shout at my mother. I shout at Less Attractive. And, to cap it all, I shout at my girlfriends. They keep ringing up and being nice, which for some reason I find incredibly annoying.

And I'm having hot flushes. The first time it happens it takes me a little by surprise. I am sitting in the hairdresser desperately having my hair dyed when I suddenly feel the need to take off all my clothes.

'This place is like a bloody sauna,' I say to the girl with the bleach, as I strip off down to my vest. 'Is there something wrong with the heating?'

'No,' she says, tweaking her neat, tight polo neck.

'There must be,' I huff, with an instant shortening of temper. 'Honestly, I don't know why I bother to come here.'

I exhale at my own reflection, only to notice that my face is scarlet and covered in a sheen of sweat. I have the skin of a boiled beetroot and whichever way I look at it – it's not bloody funny. I contemplate leaving the salon but my hair is covered in little sections of silver foil, so I sit there huffing and puffing and sweating. God, I think, shaking with anger, it's enough to make you look forward to injecting.

Fortunately, Less Attractive realizes that he is on a losing wicket and decides to take me away on holiday to start my Gonal F injections. These, the real crux of IVF, are nightly subcutaneous jabs of a female hormone that stimulates the body into producing anything up to twenty eggs in one cycle.

I'm nervous of travelling with so many needles and in fear of being pulled over for being a junkie of supermodel proportions; I get an official letter from the Lister Hospital. However, in the end, I swan through Sharm El Sheikh airport with a bag full of sharps and bottles of drugs and no one seems to bat an eyelid.

The hotel is fabulous. It is lazy luxury at its finest. It is all golf buggies, buffet suppers and unctions on terry massage tables. Just what we need. By day Less Attractive and I lie by the sea on loungers soaking up the sun in an Egyptian heat-wave. By night I am bent over the bed, squeezing the fat together on my upper thigh while he jabs away with a syringe.

It is a very odd thing, being injected by one's husband. First, I think he finds it rather upsetting. The idea of causing me pain is something that is strangely not high on his agenda. And secondly, I barely trust the man to boil a kettle, so the idea that he might get 225cc of Gonal F correctly into a syringe, without air bubbles, and inject it safely into my thigh is something of a leap of faith.

Initially we are both rather tense. The build-up to the first injection is enormous. I don't want him to do it. He doesn't want to do it. Finally we both grit our teeth. He pushes the needle in. I hardly feel it, and then there are somewhat hysterical smiles all round.

It doesn't take long before Less Attractive is so syringe-savvy he is practically taking a run-up. It seems to amuse him to ask me in a loud voice in public if it's time for my injection and he also quickly develops an unhealthy liking for 'works'. It's the flicking with his finger as he gets rid of the bubbles that particularly seems to tickle him. Meanwhile, I lie awake at night and worry about dying on small pockets of air. For me the only upside is that being pumped full of hormones obviously agrees with me. My mood improves, my skin glows, I rediscover my long-lost sense of humour. In fact I feel really rather good. Honestly, I have no idea what people complain about; this IVF thing is a blast.

5

Week three of the sniffing and injecting and I have so many eggs inside me I feel like a sturgeon. I have my first scan with Liz at the Lister Hospital. A kind and jovial woman who spends all day counting eggs and talking to nervously hysterical women, she really knows her stuff. With the use of a probe, she sorts through the black shadows on the ultra-sound screen and explains exactly how many eggs my overexcited follicles have managed to produce. I have a possible thirteen, which is apparently a good thing and means I am right on course.

And I can feel every one of them. My lower abdomen is

jam-packed with the things. Like ping-pong balls in a rubber glove, they are all jostling for space in my overcrowded groin. It is uncomfortable to sit up. It is uncomfortable to lean forward. It is uncomfortable to work at my desk. And yoga sessions are now ever so sadly out of the question. All I really want to do is lie on my sofa, sporting only the most comfy of easy-on slacks, and indulge my encyclopaedic knowledge of Australian soap opera.

Even the Gonal F injections themselves are beginning to pall. My thighs are sore and covered in little bruises. And Less Attractive has got bored with playing doctors and nurses. He can barely be bothered to flick the syringe before he makes a jab for it. It is now just part of his nighttime routine – brush teeth, inject the wife, go to bed. He becomes more jaded with each night that passes. So much so that just before I have to go into hospital to have my eggs harvested, he calls from a drinking club and announces he won't be back in time to do it at all.

Of all the injections for him to bottle out of, it would have to be this one. Pregnyl is nothing like the Gonal F jabs: it is twice the size, with twice the amount of liquid and the biggest needle I have seen outside veterinary science. Administered at exactly 11pm, thirty-six hours before harvesting, it ripens the eggs ready for collection.

I take all the bottles out of their packets and line them up on the side in kitchen. I get the syringe and needle out of their protective plastic, and stare. I really don't want to do this and Less Attractive is a right old bastard for propping up a bar in Soho. Oh lord. I inhale and fill the syringe. It's already 11.10pm. It's now or never. I grab the thing and stab it into my thigh. I push in the liquid, pull out the needle and, as blood trickles down my leg, I turn and throw up in the sink. Mission accomplished.

Less Attractive reels in drunk at about 1.30am, and instead of a cosy cuddle and chat about Wednesday's operation he gets the cold buttocks as punishment.

A day and a half later, it's 7.30am and Less Attractive and I are sitting in the waiting room, exuding jolly tension. He is terrified that he won't be able to produce a sperm sample, while I'm convinced I am going to be the teaching vagina – with a class full of students staring up my sedated women's bits, while Dr Parikh rattles around in my fallopian tubes with her pipette, extracting eggs, occasionally letting some untrained hand have a go.

The green-carpeted day room is full of other tired and anxious couples all holding hands and whispering to each other. In that very British way of politely getting on with things, we are all pretending that none of us is barren and no one knows quite why anyone else is here.

Eventually our names are called and we are moved upstairs to our room. Rather small and hot, it contains two beds divided off by a curtain. It smells of chicken soup and disinfectant. There is no relief from its clinical function; the television sets were apparently removed a while back to prevent patients from arguing over the channels.

I smile at the other couple as they walk in. The husband grimaces, the woman doesn't reciprocate. There appears to be no sisterhood in IVF. They scurry into their corner of the room and draw the curtains around them, never to be seen or heard of again.

Less Attractive and I have no idea what to do. He stands around looking worried, then he paces the room and exhales loudly – while I'm being as breezy as you can be in a backless gown without any pants on. Eventually I send him away. Being breezy is exhausting, and I can't cope with all his concerned stares. A nervous tear falls down his cheek as he waves goodbye.

But before I have time to feel really sorry for myself, they come for me. I am wheeled to the lift flat on my back on a trolley, accompanied by jovial banter and a sea of lights and smiling faces. The anaesthetist foolishly asks me what I do for a living, but I'm only halfway through plugging my list of literary oeuvres before the cold feeling creeping up my arm sends me under.

I wake up seemingly straight away to the sound of my own teeth chattering. The room is freezing, the lights are bright and my mouth is bone dry. I can hear people talking. I can make out two rows of about six women all out cold, all having been harvested. I make a moaning sound and a nurse appears. She hands me my spectacles and gives me a congratulatory pat. I'm told that they have managed to extract eight eggs. This is apparently good news.

Buoyed up by my fertile triumph, I'm trolleyed back upstairs again and filed in the small hot room without a telly, where I am left to sleep and recover. I pass out for about an hour and then have to call a nurse to accompany me to the loo. It is hospital regulations. There has to be someone on hand just to make sure they haven't pierced your bladder during the operation. My bladder seems to be working fine but there is something rather odd going on.

'Excuse me,' I say to the nurse, 'did you put something up my backside while I was out cold?'

'Not me personally,' she replies. 'But they did put painkiller up there.'

Great, I think, as I sit on my bed. The only orifices not violated, so far, by this IVF treatment are my ears.

Now that I have gone to the loo correctly and delivered my eight eggs, Dr Parikh announces that I am free to leave hospital. 'Your husband's sperm sample was also a success,' she declares, as I start to get dressed.

'At least he is good at something,' I reply.

As I stand around on the steps of the Lister waiting for Less Attractive to arrive, I feel knocked about but also slightly relieved. I can't help thinking that we are nearly there. I've grown the eggs, they have been successfully harvested, even the sperm sample went OK. It's all going to be fine.

In fact, it could almost be romantic. Less Attractive's car pulls up outside the hospital and I get in.

'Darling!' I smile, leaning across to kiss him. 'So nearly there.'

'I know,' he replies.

'Who were you thinking of when you gave your sperm sample?' I ask, staring into his eyes.

'Debbie from Dagenham,' comes his rather unexpected reply.

6

Back at home the morning after, I'm lying in bed feeling optimistic. Surely by now the worst of this IVF thing is over? I've done the injections, I've screamed through the menopause, I have lived the life of a Trappist monk, I have come out the other side and I have eight eggs in a Petri dish gently growing and dividing somewhere to prove it. I stretch and smile. Perhaps, at last, I can begin to allow myself to dream of chubby babies with blond curly hair, of sweet smiles and sticky fingers.

The telephone goes. Less Attractive is in the shower. He's been boxing in a gym that he insists on calling 'Fight Club' and is washing off the testosterone. I get out of bed and answer. It is an embryologist from the Lister Hospital and she says she has some disappointing news. I sit down slowly at my desk.

'Of the eight eggs that you produced, I'm sorry to say only two have fertilized.'

'Two?' I repeat.

'Yes, two,' she says.

'Two,' I say again, not quite comprehending how eight eggs sitting in a dish, surrounded by sperm, can bloody fail to fertilize. 'Why? How? What has gone wrong?'

'It seems that you and your husband are incompatible,' she says.

'I could have told you that a decade ago,' I reply.

'Yes, well,' she says, sounding tense. 'Look on the bright side, you only need two. Lots of people get pregnant with only two.'

As I hang up the phone, I must make some dreadful noise because Less Attractive comes running stark naked from the shower. 'What? What's wrong?' he says, standing in my office.

There is a huge crashing sound to my right, as the window cleaner, stunned by this sudden streak, brains himself on the glass. It would be amusing if I had more than two embryos. But I don't, so it's not.

Less Attractive tries to be optimistic. Two is fine. We didn't really want to freeze any spare embryos anyway.

I can't believe our bad luck. We are a quite unremarkable couple, trying to do rather a normal thing – why are we so goddam special when it comes to babies? 'What are we trying to breed here?' I say through my tears. 'Some bloody rare bird?'

I spend the afternoon with my acupuncturist, Justine, who is also beginning to take on the role of a shrink. Poor woman. But there are only so many times you can call on a girlfriend and talk solely about your vagina before even the very best of them start to tire. Justine gives me some gentle needling plus moxa (a hot burning stick that is placed close to the skin to warm the blood) and puts some golden beads in my ear à la Cherie Blair. This is all designed to help heal my operation scars and make the uterus a more blood-rich welcoming place for tomorrow's embryo transfer. She also arranges for a friend of hers, Susie Astbury, to give me a session of acupuncture after I have the embryos put back in. Studies have said that acupuncture before and after transfer increases your chances of success. And at this late stage anything that may help is, quite frankly, welcome.

The next day Less Attractive and I arrive back at the Lister with the odds firmly stacked against us. We have no choice of embryos, no embryos to freeze, and we also have to hope that the two embryos we do have survive the night and are still dividing merrily. We sit tensely in the waiting room. I am slightly tenser than he is, mainly due to the fact that I am desperate to go to the loo. Embryo transfer has to be done on a full bladder. It is something to do with the ultrasound and a lot to do with making the process just that bit more unpleasant.

Walking into the operating room, I forget that this is the first time Less Attractive has been at the stirrup end of IVF. 'Oh my God,' he says, standing with his back flat against the door, as he takes in the lights, the legs-in-the-air chair, the monitors, the rubber gloves and masks.

'Beyoncé,' he exclaims suddenly, walking over to the windowsill and picking up the latest copy of *Vogue*. 'I think we should call one of them Beyoncé, what do you think? Darling? Definitely Beyoncé . . .'

While I take off my underwear and position myself, akimbo, under a sheet, in the legs-in-the-air chair, he carries on chatting like a madman waiting to be sectioned. The only thing that shuts him up is the arrival, via a hatch in the wall, of our embryos.

'Wow,' he says.

'Wow,' I agree. They look amazing. Through a magnifying microscope on a wall-mounted television, we can see them swimming around and they are beautiful. It sounds deranged to say that a cluster of cells is beautiful, but they really are. Less Attractive and I stare open-mouthed.

'Those are our potential children,' he says, taking hold of my hand. 'Aren't they wonderful?'

'They're two and three cells,' declares Dr Parikh, through her mask. 'And they're of grade one and grade two standard.'

'Shouldn't they both be four cells at this stage?' I ask, staring between my own thighs.

'Mm,' she agrees. 'Maybe they'll divide later today.'

Then quick as a flash they disappear up Dr Parikh's long tube and, with equal speed and accuracy, she pushes the tube straight up my cervix and releases them into my womb. I inhale sharply and hold my breath as Less Attractive and I watch the two white specks sail off into the distance.

I gingerly get off the chair and put my underwear back on. Less Attractive is all pink and emotional.

'Good luck,' says Dr Parikh, as she kisses us both goodbye. 'I really hope it works for you two.'

We walk out into the street, rather overexcited. I feel pregnant for the first time in my life and I can't stop smiling.

7

There are two things you are advised to do immediately after embryo transfer. The first is to have acupuncture to help stimulate the blood supply to the uterus and the second is to stay in bed.

The first is relatively easy. I drive (rather badly) round to Susie Astbury's for some gentle prodding and burning moxa treatment, and then go straight home to bed. But the second proves almost impossible. Contrary to what Less Attractive thinks, I'm not normally one of those lazybones types prone to lounging about, taking in the delights of morning TV. In fact, I find it hard to stay in bed, particularly when I'm high as a kite on steroids.

I was told to expect side effects when taking prednisolone. It was explained to me that in order to counter the abortive nature of my NK cells I would have to take steroids, and I might perhaps develop a bit of a moon face and an increased fondness for food. But it isn't food I'm hankering after, it's filing. The drugs have made me so Miss Moneypenny efficient that, instead of staying in bed, all I want to do is get organized. Really organized. Amazingly, I'm so obsessed with admin that in the early post-transfer days I manage to do my VAT, fill in my tax forms, pay all my bills, open a bank account, apply for a credit card, tidy my office and file, file, file.

Less Attractive declares he likes his new steroid-enhanced wife and suggests that I might take them all the time. I'd seriously consider it an option were it not for the worrying blue Addiction Card I have to carry around with me announcing that 'I am on steroid treatment and should not be stopped.' Stopped from what, it doesn't actually say, but clearly I'm wired and dangerous and should be allowed to do exactly as I please. And the other great problem is I can't sleep. I lie there night after night, rolling around, tying my sheets in knots, trying to get comfortable, sighing and thinking, my brain whirring away till dawn. I call up a friend who, due to a recent illness, has also been sleepless on steroids.

'Yeah,' he confirms. 'That's 'roids all right.'

'But it's terrible,' I say.

'Have you tried listening to Enya?' comes his helpful reply.

On top of the steroids, I'm also filling myself full of progesterone, which bizarrely makes you more flatulent than a horse at full trot. It is intolerable. Designed to boost your natural progesterone levels and create a thicker womb lining, all it serves to do is make you feel even more unattractive and repellent than you do already. It also causes your lower belly to distend as all your abdominal muscles relax, making you look (somewhat ironically) three months pregnant. Oh, and it comes in the form of suppositories that you have to shove up your backside each and every morning.

All this would be bearable, if it weren't for the wait. These two weeks between embryo transfer and the pregnancy test feel like a lifetime. Having had appointments, operations, tests, hospital visits, injections and rather a whirlwind of fuss, you are left with nothing. Your diary is empty, the telephone is quiet; it's almost like being dumped. Or as any girl who has ever got married will know, it's like that weird comedown you get after being a bride. You were the centre of attention for weeks and now suddenly no one wants to know. Least of all the Lister.

Although quite what they are supposed to do, I have no idea. This is the bit where they can't do anything. No one can do anything. The science is over and now nature has to take her course. And that's what is so terrifying. Having been let down by nature for two and a half years in my pursuit of a baby, the last thing I want is for her to get involved now. Just when I look like I have all the angles covered, I have to leave the last and most important bit to chance.

And it's agony. Every twinge, every movement, every little bit of pain, sends me rushing to the loo. There are days when I allow myself to dream and think of the future. There are days when I can look pregnant women in the eye. But most of the time it's murder. I just worry, wring my hands, and keep checking my underwear, convinced that the wretched thing hasn't worked. Which, of course, is another reason not to sleep.

But so far so good. I have got to hang on in there. I'm now past the halfway point. I can see light at the end of the tunnel. I have made it through one week, embryos intact. I have a children's birthday party to go to tomorrow which I might just attend. Well, why not? That world of ice cream, jelly and bright pink fairy cakes could soon be mine. I'm one week down. Only one more to go.

8

I am so stunned I can barely move. I can only say one thing over and over again. 'It hasn't worked. It hasn't worked. It hasn't worked.' I'm whispering really. I'm standing in the sitting room, my mouth is dry, my hands and legs are shaking so much I can barely keep it together.

'What do you mean, it hasn't worked?' asks Less Attractive, looking swiftly over his Sunday newspaper.

'It hasn't worked.' I say it again. 'The IVF. It hasn't worked.'

'How do you know?' he asks, colour draining from his face as he slowly puts down the paper.

'Blood,' I say.

'Blood,' he repeats. 'But that's not supposed to happen for at least a week.'

'I know,' I wail, as I stumble forward. 'I know, I know.'

I make it to the sofa. I sit stiffly on the edge. Less Attractive comes quickly across and puts his arms around me. I don't know what I am doing. I am vaguely aware of the *Antiques Roadshow* going on in the background. Michael Aspel is admiring a table. But other than that, all I can do is rock back and forth on the sofa, pulling at my trousers. I'm freezing cold, my chest is tight, I'm finding it hard to breathe and I can't stop shaking. This is what it must be like to go into shock. 'It hasn't worked,' I say again.

'I know,' says Less Attractive.

'Why?'

Finally I start to cry. I don't make any noise but the tears still come, burning down my cheeks. They're thick and fast and there is no stopping them. Less Attractive, I think, goes to get me some water. I'm not sure what is going on. I can't really see. I look up and the world appears to have closed in. I have no sense of perspective or distance. I take a few sips of water but I don't know what to do next. The agony that I feel is so overwhelming and all-encompassing, I start scratching my hands and my legs, digging my nails in, trying to make some sort of physical pain from what I am feeling. 'Why?' I ask again. 'What did I do?'

'Nothing,' says Less Attractive. 'You didn't do anything.'

'Then why hasn't it worked?'

He doesn't know the answer. There is no answer. But there are still plenty of questions. Why me? Why this? Why can't I get pregnant when girlfriends of mine all seem to be able to do it so easily, despite drinking and smoking and having a good time? I haven't had so much as a skinny latte in seven months and still I can't get knocked up. How much of a dud must I be?

I think I'm going to be sick. I retch into my palms but nothing happens. Less Attractive rubs my back. It's actually rather annoying. But I don't know what to do, so why should he? We sit there for about half an hour. I'm so cold and shivery, my teeth start to chatter and I keep taking big gulping breaths of air. He doesn't say much. Michael Aspel carries on enthusing about some woman's china doll collection.

I really wasn't expecting this. I was so confident that I'd manage it, despite having been warned that IVF is not an exact science, that you have to do it a couple of times before they get it right. I was, of course, obviously going to be the exception to this rule. I haven't really failed at many things in my life. I didn't pass my driving test first time, but then who does? Apart from that, I have sort of managed to get and pass most things through willpower, determination and a bit of luck. We'd even bought a pregnancy-testing kit. That morning, going round Sainsbury's, I'd slipped it in among the apples. Less Attractive watched me do it. He didn't say a word. He just smiled, rather sweetly.

And now this. All that work, all those sacrifices, all that effort, all those drugs and injections and operations, all those indignities, all those people playing around with your bits, and still no baby. Not even a glimpse of one. I don't even get the excitement of doing a test, sitting in a loo, crossing my fingers, hoping for a blue line to appear.

Less Attractive suggests that I go to bed. I'm not sure what time it is, but it feels late enough to me. I'm exhausted. In fact, I'm so drained that he has to help me up the stairs. It can only be about 7.30pm. But I've had enough of today.

We get into bed and I stare at the ceiling, tears trickling down the sides of my face into my ears. Less Attractive holds my hand and asks me what I want to do.

'We'll do it again.'

'Do you think so?' he asks.

'Oh God, yes,' I say, sitting up in bed and looking at him. 'I'm not beaten. It takes a lot more than this to defeat me.'

47

'OK,' he says. 'When do you want to do it?'

'Right away,' I say. 'In fact, tomorrow I'm going straight back in there.'

9

The next morning, I find myself standing on Chelsea Bridge staring at the Lister Hospital. It's cold, raining and I'm being buffeted by the wind, but I can't actually move. All I can do is stand, my body growing increasingly rigid. I'm rooted to the spot, paralysed. Getting straight back on the IVF horse after failure, I suddenly realize, is not going to be as easy as I'd thought. I'm shaking. I feel sick. My mouth is dry, my hands cold and clammy. I don't want to go in there. The idea is not appealing. In fact, if I'm honest, I'm scared.

This takes me completely by surprise as I always thought I was a reasonably rational person, sane and sanguine in the face of difficulty. But apparently not. Standing here, looking at the red-brick building, I swear I'd sooner run stark naked round Aintree than walk back into that Assisted Conception Unit and talk about babies. I'm crying again and I'm furious with myself for being so pathetic. Come on, I say to myself, get on with it. I remember reading somewhere that if you dig your fingernails into the palms of your hands it helps you control your emotions. So I dig deep, inhale and cross the wretched bridge.

Sitting in the waiting room, surrounded by expectant faces and tense, earnest husbands fiddling with the coffee machines, I feel like letting them in on the secret that IVF doesn't work. Save your energy, I want to shout, it's not the answer to all your prayers. It's a load of old crap. It's a bloody rip-off and it only makes you miserable. But my name is called and I slope off down the corridor to Dr Parikh's office.

'Oh,' she says as I come through the door. 'I am very sad. I had hoped not to see you for a while. Four of my ladies in your group are already pregnant.'

'Oh.' I smile, sitting down. 'Just me again.'

'Sorry?'

'Am I the only one not to manage it then?' I ask.

'No.' She smiles. 'There are others.'

How many she doesn't say. But I suspect it is only a few, as the Lister has a statistically high success rate, one of the top five in the country.

'So what went wrong?' I ask.

Dr Parikh inhales. For starters my embryos were apparently rubbish. Although she has had a few pregnancies from two- and three-celled embryos, she would have preferred me to have at least one four-celled embryo for her to transfer into the womb.

'Well, why did you put them in?' I ask, quite sharply.

'Because we didn't have any other choice,' she says.

She has a point. It wasn't as if we had any other options, due to our apparent lack of compatibility. I say it's because he's from Birmingham that my refined eggs have no interest in his dodgy Bull Ring sperm. And then he always points out that so am I, so it shouldn't be too much of a problem. Either way, for some reason it seems they don't like each other very much.

But Dr Parikh has a solution. IntraCytoplasmic Sperm Injection or ICSI – a revolutionary technique in which they take hold of the sperm, cut off its tail (there is no DNA stored in the tail, it is there only to enable the sperm to swim) and inject it into the egg. Current research states that there is no increased risk of congenital abnormalities in children conceived through ICSI but they do advise that they have regular developmental assessments. However, with ICSI there is a much higher fertilization rate and therefore a better choice of embryos at the end. It seems like the perfect solution, though I can't help but think how lazy and reluctant sperm must be that they have to have their tails docked and be forced into an egg in order to get any sort of show on the road.

Dr Parikh also has other suggestions to make. She wants me to take more Gonal F – the drug that stimulates the ovaries into producing more eggs – so that we have more choice. And she also wants me to take more flatulence-inducing progesterone pessaries so that the womb lining is thicker and more alluring for the embryos after transfer.

'And we'll take it from there.' She smiles. 'Do you want to start right away?'

'Well, I don't see why not,' I say, feeling emboldened and a bit more optimistic. My situation is not totally hopeless. It seems that there are ways round my problems. Science, thankfully, has solutions where nature had clearly given up the ghost. 'What do I do now?'

'Well, I'll put you straight back on to the pill for three weeks and we'll book you in for ICSI.'

'Great,' I say, rubbing my hands. 'Here we go again.'

'Here we go again.' She smiles. 'You should give yourself a bit of a break. You know, relax. Have a glass of wine.'

'A glass of wine?' My mouth is watering.

'Oh yes,' she says. 'You should certainly allow yourself a glass or two of wine. Nothing excessive,' she adds.

I'm afraid I don't hear the last bit. Two days later, I am propping up the bar of the Electric House on Portobello Road, drinking Cosmopolitan cocktails like they are going out of fashion (which of course they are). They are not wine and neither am I being abstemious, but I don't care. It is a relief to join the human race again and, for one night only, not have to think about trying to make babies.

In retrospect, I should have taken a step back at this point. I was really holding on to the lintel of sanity by my fingertips, ready to fall off at any moment. My desire to get pregnant was so powerful and so all-encompassing that everything else paled into insignificance.

My relationship with Less Attractive was really quite strained. Poor bloke. My mood swings were huge and my ability to cope with anything other than the pursuit of a baby was non-existent. I remember getting me to go shopping for something as un-taxing as supper was an arduous task punctuated with a whole lot of attitude and a long litany of sighs. My friends tell me now that there were times when they dreaded me telephoning. They had had it with the endless fraught conversations about my vagina. One need only know so much about someone else's reproductive system. But then again, what else was I supposed to do? There aren't that many people you can lean on. Less Attractive's legs were bowing under my not insubstantial weight. My sister was hoarse from chatting and my mother was too upset about it all to take much of the strain. She was suffering from some weird delusion that it was all her fault. That she was being punished for something she had done.

And that's the problem with this whole fertility game: it

becomes so intensely personal that you lose sight of everyone else around you. I could think only of myself. My sister got engaged and one of my best friends got pregnant with her second baby. And I'm afraid my reaction to them both was pretty joyless. My pregnant friend was greeted with a fairly stony silence, a lemon-sucking smile and a tight-lipped 'well done' down the telephone. My sister, on the other hand, was simply warned that if she got pregnant before me, I'd bloody kill her.

In reality, what I needed was a few months off to rediscover the joy of living, to realize that the world didn't revolve around me, my front bottom and my quest for the pitter-patter of tiny feet. But instead of being logical, I raised my bloody-minded head, gritted my teeth, shoved my elbows out and battled on. This time, however, I went all alternative.

10

To say that I am broadening my horizons for this second round of IVF is something of an understatement. In fact, since science hasn't done the trick, I have now decided that, rather like a lush at the bar, I am open to any offers, no matter how weird and wonderful they appear. Anything in any shape, packet, pill or form has got to be worth a try, at least once.

And if you're infertile, the choice is endless. Raise your head above the parapet, put the word out on the matevine that you're interested in alternative and there's no end of strange stuff out there. I've had recommendations of faith healers, psychic healers, Chinese doctors, witch doctors, herbalists, masseurs, reflexologists, ayurvedic dieticians and some woman who talks to vaginas in north London. Plus more acupuncturists than you can shake a thin needle at. And they are all, apparently, capable of miracles. Each and every one of them comes with a life-changing story attached. They can magic ovaries out of hats, conjure children from nowhere and make the barren breed. It's a wonder that the Lister Hospital is in business at all.

Flicking through the numbers and the leaflets, I decide that there are a couple of things that are non-negotiable. First is my acupuncturist – Justine – whom I love, who really is marvellous and who I wouldn't change for anyone, no matter how much of a witch doctor they are purported to be. And secondly, I have reached the ripe old age of thirty-six without having a conversation with my vagina and I am not about to start. Everything else, I am prepared to take a punt on.

The first thing I try is the metamorphic technique, performed by Audrey Pasternak, who is on all the lists of top alternative therapy practitioners in the UK. A relative of reflexology, the metamorphic technique is based on the idea that there is such a thing as 'cell memory' and that cells carry past traumas, like a difficult birth, around with them. These memories, however, can be removed by rubbing the inner side of the feet. Not only do I know Audrey's daughter, but I also have some friends who swear by this technique, so I have to admit I'm quite excited by the time I arrive at her home near a wooded stream just outside Marlow.

I walk into her gorgeous cottage. The place is charming and she is much less floaty, diaphanous and alternative than I expect. In fact she looks quite normal and appears totally sane. She asks me to take my shoes off. I'm embarrassed at the state of my feet, which last saw anything resembling love, care and attention five months ago. She props one of my hooves on her lap and starts to rub. I don't know where to look or what to do. Do I gaze at the view? Fall asleep? Do I lie there and think of babies? No idea. Eventually I resort to what I always do when I'm feeling nervous. I chat. We chat about her dogs, the house, and a bit about babies. I cry a bit. She keeps on rubbing. I offload a bit more. She doesn't seem to mind. Then, just as I am about to bore myself, talking about myself, the treatment is over. We kiss each other goodbye, she wishes me luck and I drive back to London, feeling exhausted. I sleep for the rest of the afternoon.

Question is, am I finally relaxing after trauma has been brushed out of me? Or am I simply knackered after a long drive and an hour's conversation? Given that it is a three-hour round trip and she has a two-month waiting list at the Life Centre (her London practice), I decide it is too far to go every week for something that I don't quite understand.

Closer to home and easier to get one's head around is Zeta West – the queen of the baby scene. Written up in all the girls' glossies, she has attended at the birthing bedside of numerous celebrities including Kate Winslet and Cate Blanchett. She has a very smart set-up on Harley Street and clearly knows her stuff. The first thing she says to me as I walk into her office, crammed with silver-framed photos of famous people and their offspring, is that I should stop eating crisps. A very perceptive statement that is made even more galling by the fact that 'crisps' was my response to the 'What could I not live without?' question on her pre-appointment form. A form, I hasten to add, I have yet to give her.

'But I love crisps,' I say.

'I can tell,' she replies. 'You have water retention all over your face.'

Not something else to worry about, I think, as I sit down. Gut, backside and now facial water retention. What's next? Well, apparently lots of things. My diet must be changed again. More Omega 3 oils to help fight my NK cells. More protein to help with egg-making. And much less salt.

Alcohol, cigarettes and fun are obviously out of the window. In fact, the only joy on the horizon is that she recommends I cut down on my exercise. The body can't cope with so much egg-making if it has a step class and yoga to deal with as well. Oh, and while I'm about it she suggests I have some manual lymphatic drainage and some hypnotherapy visualization – whatever either of those are. Really, it's enough to make you take to your bed for a lie-down – with a fertility crystal under your pillow, of course.

11

So I take Zeta's advice and book some appointments in her salon. I am also, I should point out, back on the sniffing hormones. The ones that you shove up your nose twice a day, every day, and that send you screaming through the menopause. Maybe I'm imagining things but second time around they feel much worse. Perhaps I should have thought twice, waited a month or so for my hormones to settle down, before I started on this rather unpleasant road again. All I know is that I'm absolutely livid. More livid than I have ever been in my entire life, and everyone is feeling the heat.

Last time I took Synarel I vaguely remember hot-flushing

my face off in the hairdresser's and generally being quite batey. Again I have the usual headache from Dante's Final Circle that numbs the whole right side of my face, and this inner boiling anger that just won't go away. All it takes is the slightest inconvenience, the smallest irritation, and I explode.

Which brings me to the first of Zeta West's suggestions – the lymphatic draining massage. Now I know massages are supposed to be deliciously relaxing things, but you try telling this to a rabid bitch who is going through a chemically induced menopause. I can only hope that the poor woman pawing and patting me took it all in her stride. She didn't seem to mind that I lay rigid on her bed, with my shoes defiantly on, barking questions like 'Can't you do it a bit harder?' and 'How much longer will you be?' from underneath my white fluffy towel. And then when she started tapping the flesh either side of my nose to release all that facial water retention I have accrued through too many cheese and onion crisps, I actually sighed in her face and announced I had to leave, as I had a plumber arriving at home any minute NOW!

Poor old Less Attractive is not having much fun either. One of the things that seem to cause my inner anger to boil over is cooking. As a result he is in takeaway hell. Or more specifically sushi hell. Which is bad on two fronts. First because it is so expensive and we are not, to put it mildly, in our first fiscal flush as we're haemorrhaging cash trying to achieve something that everyone else manages to do for free. And secondly, if he complains, I accuse him of being selfish, as I am only eating raw fish now because I am not allowed to eat it when/if I get pregnant. No wonder then that he is having a lot of business suppers out these days and has suddenly discovered that he needs to spend a few weeks working in Ireland.

Left to my own devices and with no target for temper tantrums, my anger dissipates in mad bouts of random crying. I cry when I wake up. I cry when I try to do some work. I cry when I go round Sainsbury's. I cry when I visit my acupuncturist. I cry when my mother calls. I cry when my sister calls. I cry when my editor calls. I cry when I watch *EastEnders*. I cry when some sportsman does something brave and victorious on the TV. And I really cry when I crash my car into the back of one driven by a man who seems very unreasonable indeed. But I cry most of all every night as I inject myself with 300cc of Gonal F.

With Less Attractive releasing his inner artist in Ireland, the injecting hormones part of the IVF treatment has fallen to me. Last time he rather enjoyed giving me a dose before bedtime. This time, however, sitting on my bed on my own, things aren't nearly so witty. The injection itself isn't that painful. It's just that the popping sound of the needle breaking the skin makes me feel sick. It is also more difficult to inject yourself in different places. After a couple of days the fat saddlebag on my right thigh is beginning to feel really quite sore.

So when my lovely friend Sebastian takes pity on me and invites me down to his house in the country for the weekend, I gratefully accept but with one proviso – that someone else does the injecting for a change. On the Friday night there is a drawing of straws and a friend called Gregor gets the call. He has half a bottle of red wine to steady his nerves.

'Right,' he says, exhaling loudly at his own bravery as he picks up the needle. 'How much of the stuff do you want in here?'

'Three hundred,' I say.

'Three hundred,' he confirms, closing one eye, as he sticks the needle in the bottle of liquid and draws it in. 'Check. Three hundred it is.'

'Good,' I say, offering him a freshly squeezed piece of thigh. 'Ready?'

'Ready, yes, oh no, hang on a sec,' he says suddenly. 'I haven't done the tapping thing.'

'There's really . . .'

'Air bubbles,' he nods wisely, as he holds the syringe up to the light. 'You must tap.'

'Ready?' I say.

'Ready,' he agrees and pushes the needle into my thigh. 'Sorry, sorry, sorry,' he mutters, forcing in the liquid.

'It's fine.'

'All finished,' he announces, with a big fat grin on his face as he looks up from my thigh. 'Oh,' he says, his eyes shining with delight. 'That's great. Can I do it again tomorrow?'

And for the first time in a while I start to laugh.

12

I'm not sure if my body is exhausted after the first attempt or if it is just one of those things. Either way, when I go for a follicle scan with Liz to count how many eggs I've managed to produce, the number is worryingly low. Egg counting is not an exact science, but last time, like some superannuated hen, I managed to produce a healthy clutch of eight, and this time I can boast only a miserly five.

Five is not a disaster. I know of a girlfriend who produced only one egg and now has a lovely son, but it does not exactly give you room for manoeuvre or any great opportunity for choice. It is also enough to make anyone who has been injecting their own thighs for two weeks collapse into a weeping heap on the steps of the Lister Hospital. Especially after my fifteenth call that morning to Less Attractive (still filming in Ireland) yet again goes straight to answering machine.

Word of advice to anyone who is thinking about going down this rocky, hormone hell of an IVF path: it should not be attempted alone. I know there are hundreds of people who do go solo. I've heard of a woman who did all the drugs on her own, then called her husband back from abroad, only for him to deliver his sperm sample in the loos at Heathrow, hand the pot over to a waiting nurse and catch the next plane out again. By all accounts she got pregnant. I wonder if they are still married? Not that Less Attractive and I are anywhere near the divorce courts just yet, but I know he feels guilty about having to work while I am mainlining hormones and I have to say I am doing very little to assuage it. My reactions to events are so violent and instant, I have to share them with someone, even if they are hundreds of miles away with their head down a lens and incapable of doing anything about it.

The dearth of eggs is, however, fixable. Well, perhaps not entirely fixable but you can, according to Zeta West, optimize egg-growing conditions by eating plenty of protein, knocking back lots of Omega 3 and getting as much rest as possible. So

I cancel a weekend trip to the country with a girlfriend and go to bed with a roast chicken and plates of smoked mackerel and watercress. I read rubbish magazines and watch plenty of soppy films and when I go back for another scan on Monday morning it turns out I have produced another egg. Not bad for a weekend's work. I have to say that I am a tiny bit proud of myself. I phone Less Attractive's answering machine to give it the good news.

With only three days to go until harvesting, I am beginning to feel a lot more nervous. Thing is, I know what I am letting myself in for this time and no longer have blissful ignorance to protect me. So in order to calm my mind as well as deal with my operation issues (I keep having nightmares about various celebrities – Eminem, Russell Crowe, Dale Winton – all sitting in armchairs staring right between my legs, having in-depth conversations about my bits) I take Zeta West up on her offer of some clinical hypnotherapy with therapist Maureen Kiely. I spare her my celebrity vagina hell story but do go on to explain that, rather like being kicked in the teeth, it is quite difficult to persuade yourself to go through something so traumatic a second time. Especially when it is your body's natural and sensible inclination to gather up the back-less green gown and make for the hills. She agrees and says that not only has she various tried and tested methods to help me deal with the fear and stress of what is about to happen, but that she can also try to help 'turn down' or reduce my NK cell count. I have to say that I am a little nervous and somewhat dubious when I walk into her small sunlit office and lie back on the shrink sofa, closing my eyes.

Maureen starts to talk in one of those voices that trail off at the end of a sentence. She visually directs me down a long, long path into my subconscious. I am trying hard but the only problem is that when we arrive there my subconscious proves to be rather self-conscious, and every time she makes suggestions to me – walking along a beach, going into the sea, walking along another path into a secret garden – my brain tries to comply, gets embarrassed and starts wondering what on earth it is doing this for.

We also seem to have a difference of opinion when it comes to horticulture. When asked to enter my secret garden, I happily waft through the gates, past the banks of roses, and head off towards the water feature. Maureen then suggests that we start to do some cultivating. It suddenly becomes apparent that she is thinking 'back garden' and I'm in Versailles. She asks me to get in there and really start digging, while I had been standing there, trug in hand, directing staff with a swift wave of my suede glove. The same thing happens with the beach. She's in Brighton picking up shells and I'm in the Maldives looking for turtles. No wonder I'm always so broke, I think as I lie there, I've got a subconscious that thinks it's married to Roman Abramovich. It goes a long way towards explaining why I am always out shopping for shoes.

But having said all that, when I leave the room I feel the session has worked. Maureen has made me go from tense and slightly aggressive to feeling extremely calm and even a bit mellow. I've visualized my NK cells as bright red tulips that I can now turn off at will. And I also don't feel so apprehensive about the imminent harvesting. In fact, I could almost be in a good mood. Less Attractive comes home tonight. Wonder if I shall impress him with how I am taking this whole IVF thing in my very relaxed stride?

13

Thirty-six hours before egg harvesting and Less Attractive bounds in through the front door. He is sweetness and light, full of smiles and apologies for having left me alone with my hormones and syringes for two weeks. Or ten days, as he keeps on pointing out. He comes bearing placatory packets of Irish smoked salmon and even offers to administer the final Ovitrelle injection, which helps the eggs to mature before collection, by way of grovelling penance.

I, of course, am having none of this. For not only is one injection in the final furlong far too late, but I have become such a dab hand at self-administering that his cack-handed efforts with the phials and works are far too slow and irritating for me to deal with. And after a few minutes of him flicking the needle and steeling himself for jabbing, I snatch the syringe out of his hands and stab my thigh myself. It kills, and it serves me right. I had forgotten that this was the big, bad painful one and, as blood once again runs down the side of my leg, I rather annoyingly have only myself to blame.

Wednesday morning at 7.30am and we are sitting in the foyer at the Lister Hospital pretending to be old hands. Less Attractive is nowhere near as garrulous as during his last harvesting sortie. This time he seems fascinated by the business section of a two-day-old newspaper that he finds curling on the sofa – while I just sit there, quietly praying that we get enough eggs and that more than two of them can get their act together to fertilize this time.

After about ten minutes of waiting, we are taken upstairs to the same blue room and the same corner bed as before. Is this a good omen? Or a bad one? I can't make up my mind. Less Attractive is less concerned with omenism than onanism. Will the exhausting film shoot in Ireland take its toll? Will Debbie from Dagenham do it for him second time around? Or will some other crispy-paged lovely have to suffice? This morning he has downed more zinc than a Galloway oyster and he is so on edge all he can do is pace up and down the hospital room like a caged stallion. Honestly, what a fuss. Like it can be that difficult? He's only being asked to do what teenage boys pull off about three times a day. But I can't not be sympathetic. It would be too awful to come this far and have to go home because he can't come at all. Eventually, he gets called off to commune with his lady mag and make his deposit. Even the couple on the next-door bed sigh with relief.

Only a few minutes later and it is my turn. I remember the routine. A short pantless stroll down the corridor in my back-less gown plus dressing gown. A brief journey in the lift down to the basement. A hop on to the bed. And a huge injection of cold passing-out fluid in the back of my left hand. I barely have time to re-bore the nurse with my glittering literary career before I am flat out ready for Dr Parikh to get extract-ing. Seemingly no seconds later, I wake up, teeth chattering like I've just been pulled out of an ice-covered Thames, to be greeted by the news that not only have they collected six perfect eggs but that Less Attractive has also managed to perform. I am wheeled upstairs and have a tuna sandwich and chicken soup to celebrate.

Back home again and I spend a tense afternoon with Richard and Judy, uncomfortably tucked up in bed worrying about fertilization. Wouldn't it be great to have more than two? Wouldn't it be great to have a choice? Just a small bit of luck right now would make all the difference in the world.

Next day we get the early morning call from the embryologist at the Lister. It's good news, she says. Of the six eggs that were collected yesterday, five have fertilized. Five! I can't believe it. I love ICSI. I yell the good news to Less Attractive, who is soaping himself down in the shower.

'We've got five,' I shout.

'That's brilliant,' he shouts back.

We have a choice! We have options! Hell, we could even freeze a couple if we were feeling profligate! Things are really looking up. For the first time in a while I feel that this pregnancy thing may be within my grasp.

'It's very good news,' repeats the embryologist down the line. 'I see you have three days before transfer. Fingers crossed they keep on dividing.' Fingers crossed indeed.

14

Less Attractive and I arrive at the Lister Hospital full of hope and excitement. It is three days after harvesting and time for two of my five embryos to be transferred back into the womb. We have left it an incubation day longer than we did last time, in the hope that not only will the embryos be more advanced but it will also be easier to sort the merrily dividing wheat from the dud two-celled chaff.

We take up our usual positions in the waiting room. Less Attractive leafs through an old *Woman's Own* and tries to appear calm, while I attempt to look as relaxed as I can with a bladder full to bursting. There is a knack to the water thing and I clearly haven't got it. If your transfer is at 11am you are advised to drink a couple of pints of water at 10.15, as it takes about forty-five minutes for the water to work its way through your system. However, if there is a delay and you have to sit around waiting, legs crossed, for an hour then, of course, you are stuffed. When you have to go, you have to go, and then you have to start the whole drinking process all over again.

I am on my second loo break and seventh pint of water when we are eventually called in. I remove my underwear and position myself in the legs-in-the-air chair with as much dignity as one can in front of one's own husband. He pretends to look the other way, but I can see that he is watching out of the corner of his eye. As soon as I have modestly covered my bits with the green cloth he turns round, grabs hold of my left hand and gets chatting.

'Here we are again,' he says. 'If at first you don't succeed,' he continues. 'Second time lucky.'

The nurse laughs. He can't stop talking and I just wish Dr Parikh would get on with it before I pee all over her chair.

She stands between my thighs and, through her mask, announces that the news from the embryologist's hatch is good. 'You have two very good embryos,' she says. 'Would you like to see them?'

We both nod as the camera zooms in on our babies.

'Can you see?' she asks, as their blown-up image appears on the TV screen in the corner of the room. 'They are nine and ten cells each and both grade one.'

'Nine and ten cells,' I repeat.

'Grade one,' says Less Attractive.

'That's the biggest we've ever made,' I say.

We are both slightly overcome by the moment. I feel his hand squeeze mine. I squeeze his right back. I can't look him in the eye because I know I'll cry.

A minute later Dr Parikh is cranking me open with her squeaking speculum. She approaches the hatch with a long thin tube the length of my forearm. She sucks our embryos out of their Petri dish and then inserts the tube right through my cervix. It is not a pleasant experience. Less Attractive is glued to the monitor, waiting to watch his babies launch off into the sunset. Dr Parikh releases the embryos and everyone else but me sees them sail away into my womb.

'There,' says Less Attractive, pointing.

'You're in the way,' I say.

'Well, they've gone now, you've missed it,' he replies. 'But they definitely went.'

Although there are those who say that you can go back to work and carry on as normal after transfer – after all, most women don't know they are pregnant at this stage, so why should you change your behaviour? – I am, despite my failing before, still of the lie down, have acupuncture and take it as easy as possible school of thought. I think that anything you can do to make it easier for those embryos to hang around the better. So Susie Astbury, who performed the acupuncture last time also, comes to my house this time, and administers the briefest of needle treatments plus some blood-warming moxa to the kidney points in my feet. I take another snooze while trying to turn down my tulip NK cells and have welcoming, baby-growing thoughts.

Now, of course, all I have to do is pop a few pills and pessaries and wait. Even though I have been there before, it doesn't feel any better, in fact it probably feels worse. The two weeks seem like two months. The agony of not knowing is eternal. And last time the agony of finding out was worse. I have to admit that I am really and truly scared. So many hopes and dreams are all tied up in what is happening inside me and I have no control over the outcome. Unlike before, when I thought I'd be able to cope valiantly with failure, I now know the terrible pain when it happens. It's got to work this time. It damn well has to. I just don't know if I can go through that hell all over again.

15

I think I'm going a little bit crazy. Having spent the first three days post embryo transfer lounging around like a diaphanous dowager duchess snacking on delicate fancies such as Tangy Cheese Doritos, I have now gone into some sort of psychotic steroid-induced overdrive. I can't sleep, I can't relax, I can't watch TV and I just can't stop organizing things.

I remember this from the first time round. Instead of gently sprouting facial hair, developing a sudden fondness for shot-putting and eating all the pies, my reaction to the steroid prednisolone is to get all high and racy and keen. Less Attractive is thrilled and endeavours to capitalize on his new super-assistant wife more than he did last time, giving me all the little jobs he hates. All the films that we haven't had developed, all the pictures we need framing, the chairs that need cleaning, the shower that needs fixing, the heating that needs sorting, the letters that need writing: he offloads them all on to me. 'I'd forgotten how useful you are on steroids,' he says, as he delegates yet another small, annoying task that is definitely beneath him.

But that's not to say that it is all good DIY-juggling on the steroid front. Cross my path or get in my way when I am riding a steroid trip and you are likely to encounter some very serious 'roid rage. Vaguely cut up by a car the other day, on my way to my acupuncturist, I start flashing my lights and flicking V signs so aggressively that the man gets out of his vehicle and strides equally aggressively towards me. Unfortunately for him, a passing police van, having witnessed only the later part of the encounter, immediately stops and pulls him over, while I sail on by, still extending my middle finger.

As if all this new-found aggression wasn't weird enough, I am on double the progesterone pessaries that I had before, so I have double, possibly triple, the flatulence. It can be really unpleasant to spend any time with me. Particularly at night. Were it not for the large windows we have in our bedroom, I could be accused of slowly gassing both Less Attractive and myself to death.

The logical reaction to mood swings, manic behaviour and constant farting would be to lie low and think warm pregnant thoughts towards the two embryos sitting in my womb. The illogical would be to throw a dinner party.

I know that embracing my inner Nigella, cooking monkfish for ten and making orange Florentines is a displacement activity for worrying about what is going to happen if this round of IVF fails, but I just can't stop myself. Somehow sifting icing sugar and rolling out Parma ham seems more productive than sitting on the sofa, conscious of every twitch your stomach makes, dreading every trip to the loo.

So I forge ahead with my culinary therapy and the dinner itself is not too much of a disaster. Everyone seems to enjoy themselves, the food is edible and I make only seven swift gas breaks before pudding. More importantly I have a heart-to-heart with a girlfriend who has also done IVF (one round, one egg, one beautiful baby girl). She tells me she was so mad during the two weeks after embryo transfer that she had to leave town, and sit and drink wine and chain smoke in some country retreat, crying and wailing, convinced that the whole thing was never going to work. Suddenly my flatulent dinner party doesn't seem so insane after all.

As everyone weaves their way home, just after two, I sit down and congratulate myself on a week well done. I have one more week to go before I will know if all this hell has been worth it. But I still have to get through the weekend.

For some reason Sunday night is starting to loom large on the horizon. It was, after all, at 6pm on Sunday that I lost the last two embryos. Day nine of the treatment is obviously some sort of sticking point for me. Did I lose the last babies because they were only two and three cells when they were transferred? Or did they just fail to implant into the side of the womb? Or did my natural killer cells simply get the better of them? Did my body turn on itself and see off the two lives that were growing inside me? No one knows, not even the doctors at the Lister Hospital.

But I have to say I've got a growing feeling of dread. Sunday is D-day. Sunday is the difficult one. Get through Sunday and I might just make it. Get through Sunday and I might be properly pregnant. Just how difficult can it be to get to the end of the *Antiques Roadshow*?

16

Well, impossible, as it turns out. The same day, the same time, even while watching the same wretched television programme. I go to the loo only to discover that six weeks of pills, injections, operations and gentle cultivation of two embryos have yet again come to nought. Sitting there, head in my hands, I am distraught, but for some reason I'm not surprised. Perhaps I'm resigned to this? Perhaps I'm past believing I can do this at all? Perhaps I shall never be a mother?

Walking back into the sitting room, it's the expression on Less Attractive's face that I cannot bear. It crumples with disappointment as I tell him. His shoulders collapse. His whole body deflates. He looks at me in total disbelief and despair.

'But I thought we'd done it this time,' he says.

'I know,' I reply. 'But apparently someone up there has other ideas.'

'But the embryos were so much bigger than last time. So much better.'

'Well, apparently,' I say, 'it wasn't enough.'

It never seems to be enough.

I sit back down on the sofa and start to cry. Great sobs of misery leap forth from the very pit of my stomach. Less Attractive sits there with his arm around me, kissing the top of my head. I don't know what I am crying for most. The babies I don't have. The life I won't have. Or the great void of nothingness that has just opened up before me. All I know is that this is hell, and it's fuelled by raging hormones and gallons of self-pity.

That night I hardly sleep. I toss, turn, cry. I lie there in the dark, staring at the ceiling, thinking of what might have been. The next day I call the Lister Hospital and, when I finally get through to Dr Parikh to tell her about my second-round failure, she thinks I'm joking.

'Seriously, Imogen,' she says, 'stop messing around.'

'I'm not,' I insist for the third time.

She tells me to come in the next day just to make sure.

The following morning Dr Parikh and I are sitting in her office waiting for Less Attractive to arrive. He is late. He keeps calling and saying that he is on his way. I keep telling him not to worry, all the while wanting to punch his bastard TV-executive lights out. This has to be one of the worst days of my life and he's off making telly. It's nice to see he has his priorities sorted.

Dr Parikh is still expressing so much surprise at my losing what to everyone seemed to be perfect embryos that she asks if she can take a blood test. Just as she returns from slipping my sample through the lab hatch, Less Attractive steams into the room. He's hot, he's sweating and his bright pink face is still attached to his mobile phone. He is making the cavalry-has-arrived noises and I rather wish he'd just piss off out of here and leave me alone.

'Have I missed anything?' he asks, exhaling and adjusting his suit.

'No,' I say. 'We've just been sitting here waiting for your marvellousness to make it.'

'Well, we'd better get on with it,' he quips, shooting me a not-in-public look.

Dr Parikh thankfully ignores the enormous cloud of tension

that now engulfs her office and goes on to talk through the other options available to us. To be honest, I can barely be bothered to listen. After all, what is the point? If I can't keep two perfect embryos, what real chance have I got? She talks about more ICSI, more progesterone injections to keep the embryos in there. She talks about having them genetically tested, assisted hatching, incubation until they are blastocysts (i.e. five days old and ready to implant into the womb) and then finally she suggests I have blood transfusions.

'IVIG,' she says. 'It's basically a gamma globulin transfusion which gets rid of your natural killer cells. You'd need one before harvesting, one before transfer and a couple more.'

'What, a total change of blood?' I say.

'Well, not exactly,' she replies. 'But we have done it once before and the woman is pregnant.'

'You're suggesting a process you have only done once?' I say.

'It's been done very effectively elsewhere.'

While I sit there contemplating the full rock-and-roll of a total transfusion, her telephone rings.

'No?' she says down the line.

'No,' comes the reply.

'No,' she says, looking sympathetically across the table. No, I'm not pregnant.

'What?' asks Less Attractive, all confused.

'Nothing,' I say, sinking a bit lower into my seat.

We finally get out of Dr Parikh's office and walk outside to a waiting chauffeur-driven TV executive's car. Less Attractive switches on his phone and immediately starts to deal with the life or death calls he's missed in the last twenty minutes.

'Um,' he says, looking down, noting something terribly important on his computer diary thing. 'Where d'you want to go?'

'Home?' I suggest.

'I can't do that, I'm late as it is,' he says.

'Then right here is just fine,' I say, pointing to Sloane Square.

I get out of the car and slam the door so hard, it practically comes off in my hand. As he drives off, I flick him the Vs and give him the finger – somehow just one doesn't feel nearly aggressive enough. Then two seconds later he is back. He's instructed the chauffeur to repeat the square, and I am now being kerb-crawled by my own husband while he shouts out of his half-cocked window.

'You're being unreasonable,' he yells.

'You're a bastard!' I shout right back.

'I'm going,' he barks.

'See if I bloody care!!' I shout again, giving him the double V, double finger combination.

I have definitely had better weeks.

17

Back in the real world and things are still not going to plan. When my friends Sean and Anabel asked me, some months ago, to be godmother to their divine son, Gabriel, I had hoped to be smugly and secretly pregnant and embracing the whole motherhood thing with a glowing and graceful aplomb. Somehow being mad, sad and covered in hormonal acne was not part of the mental picture I'd painted. But as the day of reckoning approaches, there is no way I'm chickening out. You don't get asked to be a godmother very often. It is a huge honour and I'm just going to have to find a nice dress and some heavy concealer as a way of getting through it.

Anyway, I've got to stop feeling sorry for myself – for my liver's sake if nothing else. For the first couple of days after my second unsuccessful attempt at IVF I did an awful lot of drinking. Partly, I supposed, because I'd been so clean and serene for so long. Like some detoxed popstar straight out of the Priory, I'd been cigarette-, alcohol- and even wheat-free for the past two months, so the initial taste of alcohol was truly delicious. But also rather than having to deal with another failure and the ramifications of more agony, more money and more miserable trips across the bridge to the Lister Hospital, it seemed more practical to drink a few vodkas and not think about it.

Despite my vodka and tonics and my attempts not to dwell on things, I did manage to come to a conclusion. I am not going back to the Lister and I am going to give up IVF. For a while at least. Two failures back to back have proved to be rather too much. It has been hard to keep a grip on life and hard to keep anything in perspective. It has also put a hell of a strain on my marriage. Not that Less Attractive hasn't been supportive, because he has. He's had the patience of a saint on Prozac. It's just that we haven't had any fun for so long, we've almost forgotten what it's like to howl with laughter so much that your face aches and you can't stop yourself from crying.

All we have been doing, since forever, is pumping me full of injections, shelling out huge amounts of money and crossing our fingers so tightly we can't think about anything else. It really is time to join the human race again and live a little.

Or at least that is what I am thinking as I walk towards the church in my green godmother dress and inappropriately high heels. There are a lot more people in the church than I'm expecting. They are having both their children christened on the same day, which explains it. But still I didn't think I'd have to chat to so many people. I find my friend Andy and fellow Gabriel godparent. He is delightful, chatty and sweet, and then makes the huge mistake of asking me how I am. A great wave of emotion pours forth, and I make an absurd squeaking noise as I try to control it. Then, as I fail, I turn and rapidly leave the church. I stand in the courtyard, concealer and eyeliner pouring down my face. What am I crying for? Am I crying because my IVF didn't work again? Am I crying because Sean and Anabel got married a year after me and have managed to produce two children for the price of my none? Am I jealous? How ugly is that? The thought shocks me so much that I pull myself together. I scrape my make-up back up my face, pat it back into position and go to take my place in the pew.

This fertility game is not a race or a competition. I am genuinely not pacing myself against anyone else – although it is extremely hard not to be affected by everyone else's seeming ease at getting pregnant, particularly when you're so high and crazy all the time. But it doesn't do to be churlish and a lemon sucker. Just because someone else is pregnant it doesn't mean that I won't be too. Life really is too short to be tight-lipped on the telephone when they call to share their good news. One can't be negative, miserable and self-centred all the time. Otherwise friends will stop calling altogether. One falls out of the loop and becomes totally isolated. Anyway, I'm not head to head with anyone else, the only person I am really doing battle with here is me. I was delighted at the birth of both of Anabel's little boys. They are sweet and gorgeous and I am so thrilled to be asked to be Gabriel's godmother. I proudly walk towards the font, head in the air, holding my candle, ready to renounce the devil and all his devilish things.

The party afterwards is actually fun. I had planned only to stay for half an hour but end up sitting next to a delicious potato salad, with my godson on my knee, for most of the afternoon. For my own sanity's sake I stay away from the champagne, which is probably no bad thing. But I really enjoy myself. It is lovely to see old friends in such a happy context. It is also delightful not to have to think about IVF, talk about it, or deal with it in any shape or form. For the first time in a long while I am not thinking about myself and it comes as a huge relief. Perhaps there is more to life than this wretched baby-making game, after all?

18

Or perhaps there are other avenues as yet unexplored. Throughout all the misery of IVF the one constant I have had, apart from the delightful Less Attractive, is Justine Hankin. Right from the off, when I was down and depressed having just undergone two failed artificial inseminations and was fat and miserable on the world's most unpleasant fertility drug, Clomid, she had the right answers, the right attitude and some very accurate needles. So much so that I trust her opinions and judgement and when she suggests something, I listen.

It is on her advice, then, that I find myself driving to the Midsummer Clinic in Gloucestershire to meet with Chinese herbalist Michael McIntyre. A man of some repute, his clinic is situated just north of Burford in one of the quietest, most gorgeous honey-stoned villages the Cotswolds have to offer. To sit in his stunning garden packed with poppies, stocks and hollyhocks, overlooking a green valley, while waiting for my appointment is a joyful and relaxing experience in itself. But meeting Michael is something else.

I'm sure I have met nicer people before, but as I sit there, going through all my IVF attempts, failures and dashed hopes, he exudes so much compassion and empathy that I feel I want to marry the man. We go through everything – childhood psoriasis, glandular fever, malaria, typhoid, pleurisy – all the ailments I have managed to pick up on the way. We look at a fabulously gory book of skin diseases so that I can pick out my own childhood variety. And he concludes that with all that I've had to deal with, it's no wonder my immune system is out of whack.

There are no such things as natural killer cells in Chinese medicine, but Michael says my spleen is damp and my tongue all dehydrated with a frilled edge. Do I find it difficult to slake my thirst? Yes, I concur, particularly when drinking vodka. He prescribes me a pot pourri of herbs that are made up into handy little daily sachets by his assistant downstairs. He tells me to drink his herbal tea twice a day, consume less alcohol and come back and see him in six weeks.

The whole experience is so positive and uplifting that I feel I can face almost anything, which is fortunate, because my next stop this week is an appointment with the famous Mohammed Taranissi.

Mohammed Taranissi is the IVF world's shiniest star. Owner of the Assisted Reproduction and Gynaecology Centre on Upper Wimpole Street, he is quoted on the UK's Richest List and endlessly interviewed on television and radio about edicts emerging from the HFEA (Human Fertilisation and Embryology Authority). He is king of designer babies, a pioneer in NK cell treatment and has, at 40 per cent, the highest IVF success rate in the country. I suppose you could say that he runs fertility's last chance saloon. If he can't get you pregnant, no one can.

Walking into his centre in Upper Wimpole Street, I immediately realize that this is not a cosy Lister type of place. Taranissi is clearly a victim of his own success. So many barren women are awaiting his magic touch that there is standing room only in his waiting room. He also doesn't allow appointments: he runs an open surgery between 8am and 10am, which means that you have to sit and wait your turn.

I sit and wait my turn for an hour and fifteen minutes. No one talks in his dark, leather-upholstered waiting room; no one catches anyone else's eye. The only noise is the rustling of old magazines and the constant purring of the credit card machine from the admin office next door. Eventually, I'm called upstairs to wait some more on another leather chair. This time, I'm surrounded by photographs of Taranissi babies. Hung on the wall like framed trophies, they give the impression that if you sit here long enough, and feed the credit card machine generously enough, you too could leave with one of these.

Finally I am asked in for my consultation. Not with the great man himself – that would be like meeting the Wizard of Oz without going down the yellow brick road. I have to pay my dues before I'm allowed such an honour. Instead, I get a man who neither asks me my name nor bothers to say good morning, and mutters and mumbles his way through my consultation barely bothering to make eye contact. If I weren't so bloody desperate I'd walk out right now. But I am, so I stay to be humiliated some more.

'Why d'you think I lost both embryos each time on day nine after transfer?' I ask.

'I have no idea,' comes his sympathetic and engaged reply.

He reels off my suggested treatment – IVF with ICSI (£3,150), immunology screening (£780), pathology tests (£310), the IVIG plasma transfusions x 3 (£1,200 each) as well as a hysteroscopy operation (£1,160) where they look inside the womb to see if there is anything else going on. They would also like to monitor a natural cycle through a series of three to four scans (£100 each) and both Less Attractive and I have to be tested for HIV and Hepatitis B and C (£90 each test).

Welcome back to the wonderful world of IVF, I think, as I feed the machine another £130 for my initial consultation. Can't think why I ever went away.

Actually, in the end, I did take myself away. Increasingly miserable, I went back and forth to Taranissi's crowded clinic for a few weeks. I shelled out a small mortgage for the tests. I had him follow one of my cycles, while phials and phials of my blood, some fifteen in all, went back and forth across the Atlantic and they confirmed, yet again, that my immune system was too powerful and my NK cells were in full gladiator mode, and then I decided that enough was enough, and I took the whole summer off.

My little sister was getting married at my mother's place in Italy and I really wanted to enjoy her wedding. I couldn't bear the idea of being high on hormones or stuffed full of eggs or riding another deeply depressing wave of disappointment, when there was so much else going on. This was a one-off and quite frankly my thwarted attempts at getting pregnant were driving the whole family mad. My father had already suggested I give up for my own sanity's sake. My mother was trying to be positive about a life without children, jovially pointing out all the other good things that were going on, talking about all the other great things I could do. Even the ever-patient, ever-supportive Less Attractive was calling for time out. So that rather clinched it. The summer was to be relaxing, baby-quest free, and to be enjoyed. Mainly out of habit I carried on taking the herbs, downing this sweet liquorice-tasting tea three times a day, and the rest of the time I threw myself into my sister's wedding.

And when I say threw, I really mean it. Perhaps making up for the fact that I was relatively well behaved at my own nuptials, I did let my hair down somewhat. I downed rather a lot of Prosecco and rather too little prosciutto and ended up pole-dancing the marquee. Fortunately, my brother was equally badly behaved and, thinking he had morphed into Mick Jagger, stole the microphone off the band and regaled the party with his rendition of the whole of the Stones' back catalogue until two in the morning. My poor sister. I have a feeling we both let ourselves and her down, but she was very good-humoured about it all. At least I have an excuse for my madness. My brother, on the other hand, deserved all the grief he got.

My sister disappeared off on her honeymoon, the guests went home, Less Attractive went back to work and I stayed behind for some quality time with my mother. We lay around in the sun together and drank a little wine but mainly I swam, slept and ate the most delicious organic food prepared by her. It was a lovely quiet time when I recharged my batteries to prepare for the next onslaught. I had only one night of total despair brought on by a little too much sympathy and rather a lot more grappa. I wailed the house down, my make-up went south, my dignity went out of the window and my mother remained suitably sweet and supportive. Then fabulously, as in all very English households, no one mentioned a word of it the following day.

So I returned to the UK rested, relaxed and ready, braced and bolstered for round three and all that Taranissi and his hungry credit card machine could throw at me. He'd booked me in for a hysteroscopy in three weeks. It's a horrendous-sounding womb scrape operation, where they also have a good poke around with a camera to see what is going on. The halcyon days were over, I thought as I touched down at Stansted: I'd begun again in earnest.

19

I'm not sure I thought I'd ever be able to say this. For some reason, in the past two years, despite two operations and end-less jabs and pills, these three words have eluded me. But no longer. Crack open the champagne, put up the bunting – I am pregnant!

I know. Unbelievable, isn't it? No one is more shocked and stunned than I. I have no idea how it happened. I was un-assisted, un-doctored and totally drug (although not alcohol!) free. It is a normal pregnancy, achieved by the normal route. Less Attractive and I actually had sex. It was our wedding anniversary and we got rather plastered and had the sort of drunken sex where you fall off the bed and can't stop laughing, which made a huge change from the dreadful dreary 'baby sex' we'd been having every month for the past two years. Perhaps that was it?

Or maybe it's because I had genuinely given up all hope. My mind, for the first time in a while, had been on things other than babies and drugs and appointments. I'd been caught up in a whirlwind of silk, roses and confetti. I had also been worrying about the hysteroscopy operation that I'd been booked in for in ten days' time. It had been keeping me awake at night much more successfully than any of my usual barren dreams.

But perhaps the most likely reason for this amazing news is the prescription of Chinese herbs supplied by the delightful Michael McIntyre. The moment I started imbibing his not-so-foul brews, I felt better. I was significantly less depressed. My energy levels improved and I also began to lose all the hormonal fat that clung to my ribs like boiler lagging. Justine noticed that my pulse was different and my blood was pumping more vigorously. In fact, she also knew that I was pregnant way before I did. At the end of my last session she said something to me that, in retrospect, makes sense.

'Unlike you,' she said, 'I haven't given up hope of you getting pregnant naturally.'

'You're the only one,' I laughed as I got off the treatment bed.

I call her four days later to tell her what she already knows. She screams with delight and says that she felt it in my pulse.

I still can't believe it though. After all these years, all this agony and heartache, how did this happen now? Was God looking the other way for a change? Or was He finally concentrating? Did Mother Nature decide that it was about time? Did she think that I had been through enough? Or have I finally paid for whatever evil I did in a past life? Either way I can't help thinking that it is a bit of a miracle. I have become one of those urban myths I always wanted to be – the girl who gave up IVF only to get pregnant on her own. I have heard these stories a thousand times before and never thought it could be me.

The other person in total shock is Less Attractive. When I do the test on Monday morning at 6am, he is in Los Angeles. So as I stare at the blue cross on the tester stick in total disbelief, I can't share it with him. I also don't dare call him. I don't want to raise his hopes with a false alarm. I want to be certain. So at 9am I go to Dr Taranissi's clinic and get a blood test. I wait all day trying not to count my chickens. I pretend to work, but obviously achieve nothing. At 4pm they telephone to confirm the unimaginable. I am pregnant. The test is positive. I feel the rush of elation all over again. I really want to tell Less Attractive to his dear face. I want to see his expression. I want to see two years of anguish disappear. But I am also frightened that this is a one-day-only opportunity. Girls like me don't get pregnant. Just suppose this is some sort of trick, a dream even, and tomorrow the baby is not there any more. I want him to feel this joy. So I call him.

'Hi,' he answers. 'How are you?'

'I'm pregnant.'

'What?'

'I'm pregnant,' I say again.

'How?' he asks.

'I've no idea.'

'Really?' he says. 'What, properly pregnant?'

'Yes.'

'Oh my God.' His voice starts to crack and I can hear him sit down. 'You clever, clever thing.'

'Thank you,' I say. 'You're quite clever yourself.'

'No,' he says. 'You are much, much cleverer than me.'

The next day he flies home. When I answer the door that evening neither of us says anything. He just stands there with his arms open and this great big grin on his face. The long and painful wait is over and neither of us can really believe it. He giggles with joy. I fall into his arms. And we both start to cry. All our prayers have finally been answered.

20

I am still pregnant. It has been two weeks now and I can't quite believe it. I think perhaps I'm in a state of shock. After all that treatment, all those jabs, pills and operations, it seems so ironic to have achieved in one drunken moment what science failed to do so many times. I have now convinced myself I know exactly how it happened. It was a combination of acupuncture, herbs and my total lack of concentration that clinched it. Or possibly just nature giving me a chance.

However, any notion of gently sitting back, eating chocolate biscuits, watching *Richard & Judy* and letting nature, herbs and acupuncture do their worst for the next nine months is immediately dashed when I arrive at Dr Taranissi's. Getting pregnant, it seems, is really only the start of the battle: keeping it, and making sure it is OK while it's in there, is where the real art of war begins.

And drugs, it seems, are an essential weapon in the armoury. Dr Taranissi has the highest IVF success rate in the UK for a reason – he throws every single narcotic available at you. After my first appointment I leave with a prescription for prednisolone steroids, plus heparin blood-thinning injections (two a day) and 75mg of aspirin daily, as well as some of those terribly pleasant cyclogest progesterone pessaries to shove nightly up my backside.

Walking out of the door with my carrier bag of pills and pessaries, I have to admit I am a little miserable. It seems so depressing to be using all these drugs again, having done so well without them. But I know I'd be such a fool to lose the baby simply through some romantic notion that I could go it alone. After all, I hardly have a glittering track record of doing so.

Two days later and things take a slight downturn. I have another blood test – my third in a week (Taranissi's clinic is exceedingly thorough) – only to discover that I'm not producing enough progesterone. So my nightly pessaries are upgraded to large intramuscular injections that have to be plunged into my dimpled buttocks every morning.

Poor old Less Attractive doesn't know what has hit him. I know that secretly, in the past, he used rather to get off on the whole IVF jabs thing. He liked releasing his inner George Clooney, flicking the syringe like they do in *ER*. The idea of giving the wife a daily dose amused him. After all, the injections weren't too painful, the needles weren't that big and it was only a two-week stint at playing doctors and nurses.

But this is a whole new ball game. These needles are big bastards as long as an index finger. The whole length of the thing has to sink right into the bum muscle and he has to do it every morning for the next three months. It is distinctly less witty and amusing and it really hurts. I tell him it doesn't, of course. He can't see me biting the back of my hand as the needle goes in. How else am I going to get him to jab me every morning?

And if that weren't enough, he also has two heparin chasers to cope with, one in the morning and one at night. They are little ready-made syringes of evil. They hurt like hell as they go into each thigh. They also make me bruise so badly that I look like such a smacked-up junkie I have to cancel my membership of my local swimming pool. Only once do I make the mistake of appearing in my swimsuit. My bruised legs cause such a stir I can never go again.

But I don't think I should be swimming anyway. Having never been pregnant before it's difficult to know what I should or should not be doing. Everyone at the Assisted Reproduction Centre keeps telling me to 'take it easy' – although quite what that means I have no idea. Should I be in bed? Should I be horizontal at all times? Or should I just lie flat out of an afternoon? Should I go out? Is dinner dangerous? Or just podium dancing? How easy is easy? Should I be working? Of course I should be working! How else are the heparin bills (£150 a week for thirty-two weeks) going to be paid? But it is all terribly confusing. And I have a feeling that the dilemmas and questions are only just beginning.

In the meantime I think I should try to sit quietly, take my steroids, pop my aspirins, have my three jabs and get on with things. I have a scan next week. They are checking to see if there is actually anything in there. They're having a look just to make sure I haven't made the whole thing up. Oh lord! Say there isn't anything? Say I have imagined the whole thing? This is clearly going to be a very long nine months indeed.

21

Sitting in the waiting room at Dr Taranissi's, I can't help but feel awful. Surrounded by so many women all desperately wanting to have babies when you are actually pregnant makes you feel wretched and racked with guilt. I wonder if this is how many of my fecund girlfriends felt as they rubbed their bellies and watched me go through treatment after treatment? Or have my two years on the other side of the fence made me realize that crowing about such random acts of fate is not attractive in the slightest?

Either way I stay very quiet. I don't make eye contact with anyone and I keep my head down. After all, who am I to show off? All this pregnancy excitement could be a false alarm anyway.

The rustling of magazines and the ticking of the credit card machine seem to go on for ever. My hands are covered in a dank sweat; my heart is racing slightly and I can feel a headache coming on. My mouth is dry and my stomach is churning. Less Attractive has texted me twice asking for news. I wish they would hurry up. I don't know how long I can stand the tension.

I have been waiting for an hour by the time I make it to the front of the queue. Both Dr Taranissi and the less charming doctor are working today. It is potluck as to which room you go into. The woman in front of me comes out of the less charming doctor's room in floods of tears. She has obviously just received some devastating news. I feel sick as I watch her weep all the way down the stairs. What has she found out? It must have been terrible. Her whole life looks like it's been drained from her face. I am now getting really scared.

Suddenly the door to Dr Taranissi's room opens and he asks me in. This is the first time in all my visits to the clinic that I have actually had an appointment with the man himself. And I have to admit that there is something rather tantric about him. I don't know whether it is because I have heard so much about his marvellousness that I immediately think he is marvellous. But I do instantly feel relaxed and safe in his company. He looks at his notes while I talk him through my pregnancy story – the failed IVFs and the miraculous conception – and all the while he smiles.

'Nothing surprises me about women,' he says when I have finished my tale. 'They are quite amazing.'

I get up on to the bed and he readies the probe. He warns me that he might not speak for the first couple of minutes while he tries to get his bearings, but that I shouldn't worry, it doesn't mean anything. He switches the scanner on and I hold my breath. He is silent for about thirty seconds but it seems like an age.

'Oh,' he says.

'What?' I panic.

'That's odd.'

'What's odd?' I say, my heart pounding as I strain to look at the screen.

'Well,' he says, 'here's your baby.' He points to a small white dot that is flickering on the screen. 'The flickering is the heartbeat.'

A heartbeat! A heartbeat! I've got a heartbeat. I'm afraid I start to cry. It's not a loud wail. It's just a gentle sob of relief, as if an enormous ball of tension that has been knotted in my stomach for years has finally been released.

'That's my baby,' I say, tears quietly pouring down my cheeks.

'Yes it is,' confirms Dr Taranissi, obviously used to such raw displays of emotion. 'And so is this sack over here.'

'Sorry?' I say, sitting up slightly.

'Well, it looks as though you might have twins,' he says, leaning right up close to the scanner. 'Are you sure you weren't taking fertility pills?'

'Quite sure,' I say. 'I was drug-free, just Chinese herbs and acupuncture.'

'Oh,' he says, rattling the probe around for a better angle. 'Can you move your hips a bit this way?' I shift. 'Mmm, well, I can't seem to find a heartbeat in this embryo. Can you see that it is all black? So you might well have had twins and lost one, or the egg was fertilized but never really got going at all.'

I have twins and lose one of them in the space of about fifteen seconds. I don't really know how to react to that. I am shocked, relieved and saddened all at the same time. Less Attractive, on the other hand, is just relieved. Relieved that there is a baby in there after all and rather relieved that it is only one.

'So you might have had two?' he asks, sounding puzzled from a corridor at the BBC.

'Well, at one stage, for about ten minutes possibly,' I explain, standing outside in the street with my phone.

'How amazing,' he says. 'But it's definitely just one?' He checks again.

'Definitely. And I saw the heartbeat.'

'So it's really happening?'

'It's really happening.'

'We can't get too excited,' he says, desperately trying to sound a note of caution.

'No,' I say, smiling. 'Absolutely not.'

I get into the car and stare blankly at the windscreen. I'm actually going to have a baby. I can't believe it. I've seen its heartbeat and it looked so brave and determined. This one's going all the way. I can feel it in my bones.

22

Why is it that life's great romantic moments never quite go according to plan? Perhaps it's just me, but when Less Attractive proposed I burst into tears and cried so hard that snot poured out of my nose. It pissed with rain on our wedding day, so much so that my mud-coated dress looked like I was wearing a chocolate cupcake. So why then did I think that the moment Less Attractive first saw his baby on the scan would be any different?

And it all started so well.

We turn up at my gynaecologist's office on time, and we manage to find a parking space just outside. I am secretly triumphant as the last time I'd sat in the chintzy confines of his baronial hall it had been to discuss the second artificial insemination failure and my referral to the Lister Hospital for IVF. And now here I am, pregnant, with a heartbeat, and raring to go.

Henderson is all smiles and congratulations as we walk in. Less Attractive is all man as he explains how the baby is all his own work. And I am just quietly excited.

Henderson suggests we move over to the examination bed and charges up his scanning machine. I suddenly feel that dropping my pants in front of two blokes, even if one of them is my husband, is rather an odd situation. Fortunately Less Attractive is overcome with tact and walks off to the other end of the room to 'look at the view'. He returns to find me underneath a white blanket, pants and tights in a neat pile on the floor.

Henderson readies his probe, snapping on the condom and covering it in lubricating jelly; this is not how it is supposed to happen in the movies. I am now so embarrassed, it is actually rather difficult for him to get the thing into position. So while he rattles away between my thighs, I close my eyes and hum to myself, pretending the whole thing is not happening.

Finally we are ready to go. I'm lying on the bed, Henderson

is sitting next to me in a chair and the other side of him is Less Attractive, who is staring intently at the screen.

'There it is,' says Henderson, pointing with his free hand.

'Where?' says Less Attractive, leaning forward to take a closer look at my womb.

'There. See the white thing? Flickering on and off?'

'What, the black blob?' asks Less Attractive.

'That's right. See the white thing in the black blob? That's the heartbeat.'

'Really?' says Less Attractive, all excited. 'Is that it?'

'That's your baby,' confirms Henderson.

'That's amazing,' says Less Attractive.

He turns to look at me and there are tears in his eyes. He leans forward to hold my hand. Sadly Henderson is in the way. He realizes this and leans forward. Less Attractive manages to reach round him and, as tears roll down his cheeks, he gives my hand a little squeeze. Henderson hunches further over his screen, his left hand still between my thighs. Somehow when I have imagined this scene – which I have a thousand times before – Henderson is not supposed to be there. Or maybe he is, but he hasn't got his hand up my crotch and my husband and I aren't clasping him in some sort of weird three-way bear hug. It is not quite the romantic moment I am after.

'Do you want to hear the baby's heart?' suggests Henderson from his hunched position.

'Yes, please,' says Less Attractive, letting go of Henderson and my hand.

Henderson turns up the volume on the scanner and we all sit and listen to what sounds like a small dog barking under water.

'It's very fast,' says Less Attractive.

'That's normal,' says Henderson.

'How about the other embryo sack?' I ask. 'Is it still there?'

Henderson takes another look and finds the other sack. He says there's no heartbeat, but that we shouldn't worry. Apparently, plenty of pregnancies start out with two sacks and reduce to one. It is not uncommon. It is just that most women don't get scanned this early, so they never know.

'You have a perfectly normal pregnancy,' he says. 'Don't worry.'

This is music to our ears. Having spent so long being abnormal, to be normal and average feels rather fantastic. We drive home, grinning from ear to ear, and crack open a bottle of fizzy water to celebrate.

But our joy is short-lived. That evening I get a call from Taranissi's office. The second sack is a problem. They think my natural killer cells might have sprung into action and killed one embryo already. According to my blood test results, which have been to the USA and back again, my NK cell count is way too high. The other embryo, my baby, could well be in danger. I need to have an IVIG, an intravenous immune globulin transfusion or change of white blood cells, right away.

'OK,' I say over the telephone, trying to keep calm. 'I'll try and sort out a time next week.'

'No,' says the doctor. 'I'm afraid that is not soon enough. We have booked you in at 10am tomorrow.'

23

I have never felt more sorry for myself than I do when I arrive at Mr Taranissi's Wimpole Street Clinic for my IVIG. I have been booked in so quickly I've had no time to think about what I am going to do and no time to discuss it with anyone. And, as far as the situation has been described, I have no choice in the matter either. Tell any woman that the life of her unborn child is in danger of being attacked by her own immune system and I don't know a single one who would not shell out £1,200 for a transfusion of pooled-blood products, no matter how reluctant or scared they are.

And I admit I'm both. I have no idea where this 'pooled

blood' is coming from. I have no idea what it is going to do to me. All I do know is that, when I go down into the basement for my treatment, I am made to sign some document that, as far as I can work out, appears to absolve the clinic of all responsibility should I subsequently develop HIV or mad cow disease. Not that any of these things have ever happened before, mind you; all the blood product has apparently been washed and checked and processed. Even so, I don't like signing things when I'm not entirely sure what they mean.

But the three other women I am with seem very relaxed about it. They have all been through this process before and arrive armed with books, magazines and well-stocked lunch boxes. We're going to be here for some time. An IVIG transfusion takes the best part of a day.

Each of us silently takes a trolley bed and waits our turn with the nurse. One by one, she treats us to a flush with a saline drip and fits an IV catheter into our right arms, before attaching a bottle of viscous IVIG solution so that it drips slowly into the vein.

It all feels very odd indeed. The saline is freezing cold. It goes up the vein of my right arm and around my body, making me want to shiver. The IVIG is equally strange. We have all been made to take an antihistamine before the transfusion to minimize the side effects of nausea, headaches and itching around the infusion site, but it still makes me feel light-headed and out of sorts. I lie back on my pillow and try to think about something else. There are three bottles of the stuff to get into my system and at least five hours to go. I should probably try to relax.

It doesn't take long before the stiff silence breaks. We are, after all, all girls together, all in the same boat, all doing battle with our fertility and our overactive natural killer cells. Turns out that two of the three women here are also in the early stages of pregnancy, having undergone successful IVF. The other, a pretty dark-haired girl lying next to me, is full of eggs and hormones and about to be harvested. We all smile and wish her luck. It is her fourth attempt.

The day progresses, and the more the other women tell their stories, the more spoilt and ashamed I feel. What I have been through – my two failed rounds of IVF, my double embryo problem and my enforced IVIG – pale into insignificance when I hear what they have to say.

The girl furthest from me has had three rounds of IVF, got pregnant each time and lost the baby at around six weeks. This is her fourth attempt, the first time she has done IVIG, and she is now eight weeks pregnant – so far so good. The pretty dark-haired girl is similar.

But the woman in the middle is in a league of her own. She has had eight rounds of IVF and got pregnant twice. The first she lost relatively early on in pregnancy; the second, however, was diagnosed as having such severe spina bifida that she had to have an abortion at five and a half months.

Quite how she still smiles, talks, eats or gets up in the morning I shall never know. She makes me feel truly humbled and, as I lie there, drip in my arm, it finally dawns on me that maybe I'm not so unlucky after all.

24

Having recovered from the trauma of my IVIG transfusion and the possibility that my immune system could turn on my own embryo, I am determined to put it all behind me and try to experience a few of the normal things that happen to normal people with normal pregnancies. Granted I am still on steroids, heparin injections and a huge Gestone jab in the backside every morning, but that needn't stop me from buying baby books, going into maternity shops and having food fad conversations with my girlfriends.

The first thing I do is go baby-book shopping. This is apparently no simple task. Walking into Waterstone's, I realize there are hundreds of the things cluttering up the shelves – funny ones, technical ones, earnest ones, bossy ones and totally hippy ones with terrifying close-ups of large women, legs akimbo, giving birth. It is enough to turn the strongest of stomachs, and I certainly don't have one of those at the moment. However, I purchase a small selection and return home to flick through them on the sofa, while watching daytime television, like all pregnant women are supposed to do.

It takes about half an hour for the paranoia to begin. 'By now your bump should be beginning to show.' 'At around this time a line appears down your stomach.' 'When the happy hormones kick in . . .' I don't recognize any of this. I peel myself off the sofa and check in the mirror. I'm flat-stomached, line-free and most definitely sour-faced. These books are obviously rubbish. I shove them all in a pile and forget about them.

Later that night, I notice a few are missing. I go upstairs to find Less Attractive propped up in bed, his nose in *The Rough Guide to Pregnancy and Birth*. Oh God, I think, as I brush my teeth, here we go. I've barely turned on the tap before he starts.

'Darling?' he queries.

'Yes?'

'Are you constipated?'

'Um, no,' I reply.

'Are you sure?' He smirks. 'Because it says here . . .'

'Yes, well,' I reply, getting quite batey, 'I'm not. All right? So leave it.'

'You're grossly flatulent, we all know that,' he continues, amusing only himself. 'But how's your mucus doing?'

'My what?'

'Mucus,' he says loudly, holding up the book and pointing. 'There's a bit about it here and it doesn't sound very pleasant at all.'

I march out of the bathroom, pull the book from his hand and hurl it across the room.

'Ha ha,' I say. 'Very funny.'

'I see you've lost your sense of humour.' He smiles. 'Read about that in chapter one.'

Needless to say the books are now in a Less Attractive-proof cupboard and I refer to them only when I have an important question – like when should I be buying maternity wear?

Too fat to fit comfortably into any of my usual clothes, I am also apparently too small to warrant entry into a maternity shop. Every time I venture into one of these places, the assistants either ignore me or ask me how pregnant my friend is. I am beginning to feel a bit like the lead in *Muriel's Wedding* – a woman so desperate to get married that she regularly tries on big white frocks in bridal shops. In the end, I decide that elastic bands and old jeans are probably fine, and I should wait for my pregnancy to appear less phantom before I enter Bloomin' Fabulous again.

So the only thing left is to develop some sort of food fetish.

'I'm quite mad for crisps at the moment,' I mention to a girlfriend over dinner.

'But you've always liked those,' she replies. 'That's hardly a craving.'

'I'm doing my best,' I say, as I order some prawn dumplings.

It's as if I'd asked for crack cocaine. My friend looks horrified. Prawns! Prawns are apparently a maternal no-no. They're right up there with smoking, drinking and drug abuse. As are oysters, crab, lobster, sushi, blue cheese, runny cheese, foie gras, caviar, mayonnaise, béarnaise, hollandaise and soft-boiled eggs; tuna and smoked salmon can be eaten only if they are wild, free and have had endless numbers of friends. In short, absolutely everything I love to eat is off the menu. Quite why, my pal isn't entirely sure.

'Just in case,' she says.

'In case of what?'

'I don't know,' she replies. 'But you absolutely can't.'

I take a chance on its upbringing and order the salmon. It feels rather good to have something normal to worry about.

25

Monday morning 9.05am and my mobile goes.

'Hello,' comes the voice of my gynaecologist Mr Henderson. 'Can you talk?'

I mumble something in the affirmative. 'We've got your blood test results and I'm afraid to say that there is a one-in-five chance of your baby having Down's syndrome.'

'One in five,' I say optimistically. 'That's not bad.'

'We were hoping for something over one in two hundred and fifty,' he replies.

'So it's bad,' I say.

'Well, it's not good,' he replies.

And so begins one of the worst weeks of my life.

I put down the phone and collapse into a chair. To say that I feel sick is an understatement. My legs are shaking. My whole body is shaking. My mouth goes dry. I think I might actually pass out. This has come totally out of the blue.

Only the week before, Less Attractive and I had been celebrating. We'd had the nuchal fold test, where they check for fluid at the back of the baby's neck, and it had passed. We'd seen its little kicking legs on the screen, laughed at its fat stomach and high-fived each other as we left Henderson's office. We were three months in. One more hurdle down. I even had a large glass of wine to celebrate.

And now this. I call Less Attractive at work and sob down the phone. He is amazingly brave. He says there is a four-out-of-five chance that the baby will be fine. He says if he'd had odds like that for every exam he'd ever taken he'd have been pleased. I tell him he is right. He tells me it will be OK and we decide that we should have the CVS test. Similar to an amniocentesis, a CVS (chorionic villus sampling) is performed earlier in pregnancy and they take a small amount of the placenta rather than amniotic fluid for testing. The test is nearly 100 per cent accurate but, as with all invasive procedures, there is a slim chance of miscarriage.

We make an appointment for Wednesday. For two nights I don't sleep. For two days I can think of nothing else. The stream of advice I get is endless. Don't do it. Do do it. What do the doctors know anyway? Someone actually says, 'Wouldn't it be awful if the baby was fine but you lost it anyway?' But most of my girlfriends are stars. Some of them have been through something similar. In fact, the more I speak about it, the more I discover how many babies fail the Down's syndrome test. Apparently it's the blood test that trips most of them up. 'If you pass the neck test and fail the blood you have a lot less to worry about,' explains one of my friends whose bright little girl had a one-in-ten prediction. Another who had a one in three told me not to worry at all. 'Doctors are paid to come up with statistics,' she says. 'They don't really mean that much.'

Wednesday and we go to see Mr Pranav Pandya at the Women's Ultrasound Centre in Harley Street. A CVS expert, he exudes such gentle calm that I actually feel quite relaxed as I climb up on to the bed. Before he injects my belly with local anaesthetic, he scans our baby on to the screen.

'There's the heartbeat,' he says. 'Here's your placenta and this is where I shall be going in.'

'I'm going to close my eyes,' I say. 'But just in case you think you can mess up, my husband will be watching you like a hawk.'

'That's fine.' He smiles. 'As you can see, I shall be miles away from the baby.'

Pran is as good as his word. He injects my belly, and then pushes a thin tube into my side. It pops as it goes into my womb. The baby apparently sprints off down the other end of the screen. Pran places a needle inside the tube. He then rattles the needle up and down inside the tube, inside my womb, some thirty times in order to collect his sample. The sensation is horrible. Less Attractive squeezes my hand. I bite the inside of my cheek. This is no fun at all.

And then it is over.

I return home to spend that night and the whole of the next day in bed. I forget how many times I pray not to have a miscarriage and for my baby to be all right. All I know is that I definitely bore myself and probably the Lord. Then at 5pm on Friday night, just as Pran's office is about to close for the weekend, we get the call. The nurse says that not all the cultures are back but from the data they have they can give me the all-clear. She says something along the lines that she thought I'd like to know rather than having the whole week-end to worry in. The all-clear. The all-clear. The words take a while to sink in. I am so happy, elated, excited and exhausted all I really want to do is go to sleep. It is like someone has punctured my balloon and I can finally collapse on the sofa. I feel so drained, so hollow, that I can barely call Less Attractive. But I do and he can't contain his delight. He repeats the words over and over, his voice all cracked with emotion. The hell, the worry, the agony, it all disappears and we are left feeling like we've both been hit by a truck.

'Do you mind if I go and get a little bit drunk?' he asks.

'Please!' I reply. 'Go and get absolutely plastered.'

26

Having been through the Down's syndrome trauma and come out the other side with my sanity just about intact, I have decided to think positive and try to get on with the rest of the pregnancy as normally as I can. With this in mind, I telephone around a few of my girlfriends and tentatively ask what other mothers-to-be are doing at this stage. The response is terrifying.

Have you booked your antenatal classes? Are you doing yoga? Are you having reflexology? Are you rubbing oil into places you've never heard of? Have you ordered all the baby kit? Do you want a pram? A pushchair? Are you having a maternity nurse? Are you breastfeeding? Where are you having it?

Feel free to call me thick, but I am afraid I don't have an answer to a single one of these questions. The fact that I never thought I'd get this far has, I suppose, made me terrified to plan ahead. Two weeks ago, it was touch and go if I would have the baby at all and now, as I walk in to see my GP to announce that I am, in fact, pregnant, she can't believe that I have left it this late.

'But you are nearly four months,' she says.

'I know,' I agree, rather proudly.

'Well, you won't get your first-choice hospital or even your second.' She is practically sucking her teeth. 'We'll have to see if we can squeeze you in somewhere.'

'I was wondering if there was a chance of having a private room . . .'

'Why don't we see if we can get you a hospital?' she replies brusquely.

I am eventually allotted St Mary's Paddington, which, according to those who know, is marvellous. I'm told I have landed on my feet. I am then sent a card for my first NHS antenatal appointment. Having spent the last two years sitting on Hepplewhite chairs in stucco-fronted mansions on

Harley Street, this is a rude awakening to say the least. First, I am seventy years older than anyone else. Secondly, I am the only woman not accompanied by a youth playing some sort of game on his mobile phone. And thirdly, they keep me waiting for two hours. When I do finally get to see someone, they seem less interested in the baby and more interested in my personal life. They ask me the most probing questions. Have I ever seen a social worker? Am I married? What does my husband do? Do we own or rent our house/flat? How do I plan to look after the baby? Do I have mental health problems? It's only a matter of time, I feel like saying. They take ten minutes to find the baby's heartbeat. And then they refuse to use the £1,200 of blood test results that I have brought along with me and insist on taking another seven phials of blood, saying they want to use only their own results.

As I leave, cross and frustrated, I have to smile. I never thought I would be wistful for the good old days of IVF.

Back with my to-do list and, after my late hospital entry, I decide that I should become a bit more efficient. So I book myself into an series of antenatal classes run by a woman called Christine Hill in west London, and I also arrange to interview a maternity nurse.

When the maternity nurse, Amanda, arrives, she is of

course strikingly young and strikingly on the ball. Will I be feeding on demand? Or am I a routine type of person? Bottle or breast? The questions come thick and fast and, yet again, my mouth hangs gently ajar as I fail to answer any of them. It is clear to me that I have been so obsessed with getting and staying pregnant that I've not actually thought about what I would do afterwards.

Antenatal classes are just as bad. Not only is everyone else's bump rounder, bigger and better than mine, they all seem to be so much more organized and together. They have obstetricians, they've been round their hospital of choice, they've got the car seat, the Moses basket, the mobile, the J-cloth knickers. They all already seem to know their pelvic floors from their perineums, and it's a wonder they need to turn up to classes at all.

However, as the class progresses and we sit and share our pregnancy problems so far, there is a light at the end of my own tunnel of inadequacy. One of them has been sick for months, another has backache, a third has piles, a fourth is having difficulty sleeping. Me? Apart from all my fertility problems, thousands of injections, Down's syndrome scare, constant flatulence and general foul temper, I'm absolutely fine. At last, it seems, I've got something right after all.

27

Things are going so well that Less Attractive and I are actually quite excited about our twenty-week scan. Not only will we get to have a good look at 'the Passenger', as Less Attractive is now calling our baby, but we can also be quite confident of everything being fine. After all, one of the advantages – more precisely, the only advantage – of having gone through the Down's syndrome trauma and subsequent CVS test is that we have now a genetically tested baby. So what could go wrong?

We arrive at Henderson's office for the scan. (This is my last treat to myself – to have this important scan done privately before I resign myself to the whims and queues of the NHS.) Less Attractive is all jokes and smiles and I am all pent-up anticipation. The woman warms up the scanning jelly, while I get comfortable with my belly out on the bed. The first thing we see is the head. Nice and round with what looks like a lovely straight nose and no cleft palate: the scanning woman seems pleased. Less Attractive gives my hand a squeeze and announces that the Passenger already looks like him. And we all wholeheartedly agree.

We carry on. There's a nice straight spine, ribs, lungs and a belting little heart. There are no signs of spina bifida, which is what they are principally looking for at this stage. I smile to myself. The advantage of years of IVF is that I have been using so much folic acid for so long, I could almost deal the stuff. It has surely paid dividends here. The Passenger suddenly performs a marvellous gymnastic move that concludes in a somersault and the scanner remarks on what an active little baby I have. I blush with pride.

Then, suddenly, she goes quiet. She is measuring legs and arms and long bones, clicking away with her scanner and computer, writing things down. She's stopped making polite conversation and appears to be really concentrating. My heart starts to race.

'Is there anything wrong?' I ask.

'Well,' she says, 'let's just get all the information together, shall we?'

Another five long, silent minutes later and we are sitting in Mr Henderson's office while he looks over the results.

'Your baby's arms and legs are short,' he says. 'They are off the bottom of the scale for what is considered normal growth at this stage.'

'Right. Are you trying to tell me that I am having a dwarf?' I joke, grinning at Less Attractive, sitting next to me.

'Well, we can't rule that out at this stage,' he says.

I swear to God that if I were slimmer, slicker and faster on my feet I'd have punched his smug lights out then and there. There are ways of delivering news to pregnant women and that certainly was not one of them. Without any warning or consideration, the man has just suggested I might be having a dwarf. I am so angry all I want to do is get out of his office. He starts muttering about having 'a chat' to discuss our options, and I'm afraid I just get up and go. I leave Less Attractive behind to sort out our next step, while I pace up and down outside on the landing, too furious even to say goodbye.

We drive home in total silence. Unfortunately, Less Attractive and I are quite similar. When either one of us is slightly nervous you can't shut us up. However, if we are scared witless we don't speak at all. It is a long and miserable half-hour in the car. The rain hits the windscreen. Neither of us looks at the other. Then, just as we pull into our road, I let out an enormous sigh.

'There's always panto,' I say.

'What?' he says.

'I know it's seasonal,' I say, 'but they'll always get work in panto.'

'No, you're right,' he replies, starting to laugh. 'Nothing to worry about at all.'

An hour later and we are back at the Women's Ultrasound Centre being scanned by the delightful Pran Pandya, who performed our CVS only a few weeks ago. He measures every bone in the Passenger's body and puts it all together in a chart. We then sit at his desk to discuss our options.

The baby is certainly small, he says, and both its arms and its legs are much shorter than they should be. The reasons for this are varied and complex. Either I am simply having a small baby who will plump up nicely soon after it is born. Or I have a placenta problem, which means that the baby has intra-uterine growth restriction and will probably have to come out early, although how early is anyone's guess. In which case, it will be born small and remain small for a while, but should eventually catch up. Or I am having a dwarf.

How bad the dwarfism may actually be is, again, anyone's guess. There are forms of skeletal dysplasia (or dwarfism) that are fatal. There are forms that are crippling. And there are forms that you would hardly notice at all. A lot more people have skeletal dysplasia than actually know it. There are plenty of short adults walking around who lead normal lives and no one is any the wiser.

His advice is to go home, have a glass of wine and come back again in two weeks. And, oh, try not to worry.

28

If you believe in karma then, judging by the last two weeks, I must have been a right old unpleasant piece of work at some stage in my life. For just as my baby starts to move and kick about in my belly, like some divine little butterfly preparing for take-off, so the doctors begin to talk about a termination.

In the first few days of hospital appointments following the bad twenty-week scan, the T-word comes up twice. The fact that I am pregnant enough for the baby to be on the cusp of surviving, should it decide to come out now, is an irony that passes none of us by. For an abortion to be justified at this late stage, the baby's condition is supposed to be chronic or life-threatening. Two doctors are also needed to sign the certificate to approve the operation.

However, every time the Passenger's determined little body is scanned, no one quite knows what to conclude. It is definitely small, its legs are short, but are these really reason enough for it not to be allowed to live? On these grounds alone, Kylie and Napoleon would never have seen the light of day. And who says an emperor with a great backside won't go a long way?

I have to say that I don't pause to think about it for long. After two years of fertility treatment, two failed IVF operations, a miraculous conception, jabs, pills, a total change of white blood cells and a Down's syndrome scare, it's going to take more than a couple of short thigh bones to make me give up on this little person. Less Attractive is even more resolute.

'If it's a dwarf, it's a dwarf.' He shrugs. 'It'll be my dwarf and I shall love it all the same.'

Both the doctors are, I think, a little relieved. They had offered to perform the termination but both had also refused to sign the certificate. Clearly neither of them was that keen to take the responsibility or go through with it.

Having decided that termination is not an option, Less Attractive and I spend the next week or so crossing our fingers and willing our baby to grow. The longer I manage to keep the baby and the more it grows, the better the odds against some sort of deformity. According to the doctors, babies with skeletal dysplasia present different growth curves to other babies. Instead of gently arcing as they gestate, the curve flattens out. The same goes for babies with intrauterine growth restriction or IUGR (when the placenta is not working at full throttle), which is another possible reason for my baby's reduced size.

So, on a serious growth mission, I up my fish intake and pile on the protein like some athlete training for the marathon. I start taking extra calcium, drinking pints of foul milk, eating cakes (unsurprisingly, babies like cakes) and sleeping in the afternoon. It sounds like bliss, but it is not. Being told to eat, sleep and relax is a sure-fire way to make you tense. And trying not to be tense about a situation that is exacerbated by tension only makes you all the more . . . well, tense.

There is something else to add to the mix. If my baby has IUGR then it may well have to come out early. Very early. Like in the next couple of weeks. For some reason this troubles me more than anything else. I made the stupid mistake once of watching some documentary about premature babies and what it takes to keep them alive. The images of their red-raw skin, the tubes and the possible complications like cerebral palsy have haunted me ever since. Poor old Less Attractive. Every so often, when things get a little too much, I burst into tears and mutter something irrational like. 'I don't want a red rat in a hat stuffed with tubes in a transparent perspex box.'

Two weeks later we return to Pranav Pandya at the Women's Ultrasound Centre for another growth scan. I am so worried and sick, I can hardly breathe. Will the Passenger have grown? Will it be enough? Will the chart be flat? Will it have to come out now? I can see that Less Attractive is on the verge of tears. Pran scans away in silence. He measures every bone in my baby's body. He prods and tweaks to make it kick.

'Well,' he says, 'it has grown.' Less Attractive makes a croaking sound. I don't dare look at him, in case he loses it. 'But your baby is still well below the size it should be. But it is moving along.' He tries to sound optimistic. 'The diagnosis does, however, remain the same.'

'What do you think to us going on a two-week baby-growing holiday?' Less Attractive asks suddenly.

'I think that is one of the best ideas I've heard in ages,' Pran replies.

29

As baby-growing holidays go, our sojourn at Lémuria in the Seychelles has to be one of the most perfect trips I have ever done. After all the tension, the tests, the scans and the hundred and one small-baby diagnoses, to run away and flop on a beach is the most fantastic antidote to it all.

And we really are running away. Two days before we fly we are offered an appointment with Dr Lyn Chitty, a genetics consultant who works out of the Fetal Medicine Unit at University College London Hospitals (UCLH) and is one of the top skeletal dysplasia experts in Europe. She has recently been on a sabbatical and has just, as it were, come back on to the market. In a fit of head-in-the-sand irresponsibility we turn it down, deciding it is better to spend ten days living in happy ignorance than sitting on the beach endlessly discussing her diagnosis. I explain to Less Attractive that if I really put my mind to it, I'm sure I can grow our baby back on to the charts. Some rest, some fish and a bit of sun and Lyn Chitty will find our child the most boring case to cross her desk in years. He agrees and we book ourselves an appointment for our return.

We are both rather excited when we turn up at the airport. Less Attractive has read in one of my numerous humourless books that it is important to have a hand-holder of a holiday some time during the pregnancy to remind you and your partner why you hooked up in the first place. So he is full of romantic plans that involve beach walking, massage and candlelit dinners. I, on the other hand, just want to get there.

An eleven-hour flight even when you can comfortably fit into an airline seat is not much fun at all. Add to that a large belly and a constant desire to go to the loo and you are halfway to understanding quite how unpleasant the whole experience is. Squeezed into your seat, piped into elasticated support socks, you can't even get drunk or pop knockout pills. Halfway through the flight, Less Attractive is out cold, his mouth open, catching flies, while I'm making my seventeenth trip to the loo. Needless to say, he arrives open-eyed and slightly hungover and I am puffed and bloated like I've been sitting on a bicycle pump for the last twenty-four hours.

Thank God Lémuria is heaven, otherwise this half of the hand-holder would be demanding a divorce. Set in palm groves with three beaches, three swimming pools, an eighteen-hole golf course and a Guerlain spa, Lémuria is the most luxurious resort I have ever been to. And I usually hate these sorts of places.

The preserve of newly-weds and nearly-deads, such resorts usually contrive to pleasantly lobotomize you when you arrive, making conversation minimal and decisions impossible. Normally all you are capable of doing is moving from the same lounger to the same seat for dinner, where you order the same food and have the same conversation with your new, or very old, husband or wife.

Yet Lémuria is not like that at all. It is an energizing place with great food, stunning beach walks peppered with turtles' nests and the largest presidential suite in the world. Less Attractive and I could not be happier in our de luxe villa. We lounge around all day, eating fish and cakes, occasionally launching ourselves into the turquoise sea – the only downer being that I am winter white, my ankles remain stubbornly puffed and I have made the mistake of only bringing a bikini. I haven't worn a bikini since I was fourteen. Quite why I think I can get away with it now, I can only put down to hormones.

Weirdly, Less Attractive doesn't seem to mind that a big white woman keeps following him around. In fact, he is sweet. He spends hours baby-bonding, talking to the Passenger, telling it stories and asking it to grow. And he's not the only one who takes an interest. Hotel staff and guests come up and ask me questions. Then again, if a listing iridescent beach ball in an unfortunate two-piece approached me, I might possibly have a few things to say.

Sadly the trip is over too quickly, and it is time to return to the grim realities of home. Standing at the luggage carousel waiting for our bags, I suddenly burst into tears.

'I don't want to go to hospital,' I sob. 'I don't want any more tests.'

'Listen,' says Less Attractive, taking my hand. 'The baby is bigger, you are so much bigger. You've just got to hang in there.'

'How much longer do I have to be brave?'

'Just a little bit more,' he says.

30

The day of reckoning has arrived. Less Attractive and I set off for UCLH and our meeting with the genetics specialist Lyn Chitty. We are both very quiet and very frightened indeed.

It is pouring with rain and we are wandering round the back streets of Bloomsbury looking for the entrance to a huge Victorian hospital complex. We finally find something promising and make our way to the second floor. As I stand in the lift, I feel my heart starting to race. Have I managed to grow the Passenger back on to the charts? Has our holiday made a difference? Or does our baby have a genetic disorder? Will it always be tiny? Just a few more minutes to go.

It is only as I pace around in the waiting area past the non-functioning drinks machine that the seriousness of the situation finally dawns on me. Walking up the strip-lit corridor I come across a noticeboard covered in photos of tiny newborn babies with their names and survival stories catalogued underneath: James, double lung shunt in the womb. Molly, fifteen blood transfusions in the womb. Melanie, hole in the heart . . . The list goes on and on. This is obviously a place for very sick children indeed. My stomach is churning, my hands are sweating. I can't believe that we're actually here at all.

Dr Chitty pokes her head round the office door and asks us in. There are another five people, all in white coats, also standing in the room.

'Do you mind if they observe?' she asks, charging up the scan machine. 'We're a teaching hospital.'

Less Attractive and I readily agree to the audience, and as Lyn swipes the scan over my stomach we both hold our breath.

'There's your baby,' she says, as the Passenger comes up on the screen. 'And it seems to be very happy in there, biting its own toes.'

'Its mother does that all the time,' says Less Attractive.

Some of the white coats laugh. I am too nervous to say or do anything.

'Right,' announces Dr Chitty. 'Let's get cracking.'

She starts to scan our baby. She runs the probe quickly over my gelled belly, shouting out measurements to another white-coated colleague at a computer across the room. No one else says anything. There is no murmur of approval, no sign that things are either good or bad. Every so often, the colleague at the computer clicks all the measurements into a growth curve graph and everyone silently gathers around.

'What's it looking like?' I ask, unable to bear it any more.

'Interesting,' says Lyn.

She goes on to explain that you would expect to see certain signs when scanning a baby with skeletal dysplasia. A flat rather than a round forehead. Poorly calcified, noduled or bowed long bones. A pinched ribcage. Some sort of heart problem. Poor kicking ability. And short fingers on the hand.

'Your baby,' she says, 'has none of these.'

'It doesn't?' I say, a large smile breaking across my face.

'No,' she says, 'although I haven't been able to look at the hands properly. I can't get the baby to wave at me. But everything else seems OK.'

'So it's all right?' says Less Attractive, leaning across.

'Well, it is still small,' says Lyn. 'And its long bones are short.'

'How short?' I ask.

'That is the million-dollar question,' she replies. 'Let me finish the scan and we'll see. One thing I do know,' she smiles, 'is that your child is incredibly rude.'

'Rude?' I ask.

'Yes,' she says. 'It's just yawned with boredom in my company.'

'Oh, sorry,' I say. 'Its father does that all the time.'

Ten minutes later and Less Attractive and I are sitting in the next-door consulting room awaiting Dr Chitty's verdict. She arrives with all of the Passenger's measurements printed out on a chart. She says that although our baby does not currently display the classic signs of skeletal dysplasia she cannot rule it out. The long bones are short, the arms and legs are on the fifth percentile below what would be classed as normal growth but there could be numerous reasons for this. My placenta is notched, although the blood flow to the foetus is fine. My previous fertility problems could be a contributory factor. A lot of small things could have combined to produce this result. Only time will tell. In fact, some dysplasias are so mild they are not detected until the child is two or three years old. Some are barely noticeable at all. We will only know for sure when the baby is born. And even then possibly not for a while after that.

However, the good news is that our baby is growing and the longer that this carries on, the more likely it is that we may find our way out of the woods. She wants us to come back in a month for another scan, and is going to book us into Great Ormond Street Hospital for further tests after it is born.

'That went well,' says Less Attractive as we stand in the street afterwards.

'Did it?' I reply.

'Oh yeah,' he confirms. 'Trust me. It's all going to be fine.'

31

With the cloud of doubt still hanging over our heads and looking to stay there for quite some time, Less Attractive and I resolve to try to carry on as if nothing is wrong. And normal pregnancy behaviour, as far as I can gather from all the books, involves a lot of shopping, some antenatal classes and, more interestingly, an evening session at 'daddy school'.

Breaking ourselves in gently, we start with the shopping. After all, how hard can it be to buy a pushchair, a Moses basket and some nappies? Well, if you're Less Attractive and me, it's apparently impossible. We go to Peter Jones, look at all the prams, pushchairs and buggies and start to panic. We are overawed and daunted. Who'd have thought there was so much choice? Buying baby transport is as tricky as buying a family car. Anyone (namely me) who thinks that you simply buy a thing with some wheels and hope for the best is sorely mistaken. There are whole systems available. Things that collapse. Things that don't. Things that clip on, clip off. Attachments. Accessories. The baby has to be flat. Then it sits up. And you must have a container for every occasion. Neither of us can deal with it at all. We wander around, our mouths ajar, pushing a few things, prodding a couple of others. We are racked by indecision and exhausted by boredom. So we buy some bibs, a very useful sunhat and leave.

Truth be known, it's not just cots and buggies that I find difficult. I find the whole baby retail thing rather hard to handle. Part of it is that I'm not one of nature's shoppers and I find the idea of spending so much money on someone so little rather unattractive. Part of it is also because I don't really know what stuff to buy. What's good? What's useful? Do I really need that? Or am I simply being ripped off? But mainly, I think, it is because I'm superstitious. So far things have not gone that well, and I can think of nothing worse than decking out a room only to return from hospital with no one to put in it. I keep thinking that if I don't allow myself the pleasure of buying ridiculously small clothes, then I won't be tempting fate.

There seem to be no such doubts among the women in my antenatal classes. They all seem to be plumping up nicely and discussing the delights of Bugaboos versus Mamas & Papas without an apparent care in the world. Most of them are a few weeks ahead of me in terms of gestation so perhaps they have been through their paranoid doubting period and come out the other side. Or maybe they never had these doubts in the first place. After one session I share my thoughts with the course leader, Christine Hill. Not only does she totally understand where I am coming from, she also proves to be fantastically sanguine. She says that if you lose a baby, emptying its room is the least of your worries. And I have to say, I kind of see her point.

Reassured, I sit back in her classes and try to concentrate on the joys of birth and breastfeeding. I am introduced to pumps, forceps, ventouses, episiotomies and electrical pain-relief machines. Part of me is intrigued, part of me is appalled and another part is in such denial that all I can do is look round the room and feel terribly sorry for all the other women who are going to have to go through this nightmare. Quite what I think will happen to me, I have no idea.

I think the same sort of feeling comes over Less Attractive when he turns up for his night of 'daddy school'. He is already quite verbose when we get into the car. He is cracking jokes and asking if he can leave early, which is a sure-fire sign of nerves. When we arrive at Christine's house in leafy Chiswick, things do not improve. Instead of sitting quietly, nibbling on a Pringle and sipping his one glass of Shiraz like all the other somewhat resigned-looking dads-to-be, Less Attractive knocks back three glasses of red in quick succession and then puts his hand up to ask questions.

'Um, excuse me,' he says, waving at the woman giving the class. I sink deeper into my canvas chair, hoping that the ground will swallow me up. 'When the waters break, does it hurt?'

The woman turns round.

Less Attractive whispers loudly in my ear, 'Is that a stupid question?'

'No, actually it doesn't,' says the woman taking the class.

'Oh, right,' he replies, a great big grin on his face. 'So when does it start to get really painful?' He looks round at the other dads for some sort of humorous support. They all stare at their shoes.

'Well,' says the woman. 'That all depends . . .'

161

'But on a scale of one to ten, what's the worst bit?'

'Well . . .' says the woman, refusing to be drawn. 'None of it need be that bad.'

'Oh,' says Less Attractive, sounding a little disappointed. He leans over and whispers again. 'Gas, air, drugs, the whole thing sounds easy. I don't know what all the fuss is about!'

32

It's four weeks since Less Attractive and I last visited the foetal medicine unit at University College London Hospital and I am back again for our final growth scan before the birth.

In the last month I have been popping calcium pills and drinking pints of milk in the hope that some late bone-building spurt might do the trick and the Passenger might surge back on to the chart, back to within the parameters of what is considered normal. Although I don't hold out much hope. My bump is still half the size of everyone else's in my maternity class, and with the pressure of will-my-baby-have-a-growth-problem-or-not going on I haven't exactly been able to take it easy.

But Less Attractive and I are now more or less resigned to the whole thing. I think we have heard so much doom and gloom that we have become immune. So much so that Less Attractive has decided not to come to this scan. The logic being, we'll only get more bad news that we will choose to take in our stride and then ignore.

So I am sitting on my own and staring at the photos on the wall of the terribly ill children the unit have helped into the world. Alice, double lung shunt in the womb. Tom, hole in the heart. I keep imagining our photo: 'Boris, skeletal dysplasia.' I think I'm having a boy, as does absolutely everyone else. I have done numerous ring tests, where someone strings a wedding ring on to a piece of cotton and watches it turn above your stomach bump. The ring spins one way for a girl and the other for a boy. I get a boy every time. So we are all in agreement that a small chap is on his way. Except for Less Attractive, who is holding out for a girl. In fact, he's got his fingers so tightly crossed for a girl that I actually had to take him aside and have words with him the other day, just in case his dreams don't come true.

It may seem odd that we have the most scanned baby in the

world and we still don't know the sex. But I have fought to keep it that way. Everything else about this baby has been tweaked and photographed and discussed and dissected, I want to let it keep a tiny bit of mystery. However, in the event of a boy I have been working on the name Boris. Less Attractive is not keen but has rather unhelpfully come up with no alternative. Fortunately I still have a couple of weeks to convince him.

Dr Chitty finally calls me in. This time there aren't as many people in white coats floating around the room as before. Perhaps our case is no longer so compelling? Or maybe they learned all they needed to on the previous occasion?

'Right,' says Lyn, starting up the ultrasound machine. 'Let's have a look at this little person.'

I lie staring at the ceiling, holding my breath. I now slightly regret Less Attractive not being here. I could do with someone to hold my hand. Lyn seems to be taking ages, measuring all of the Passenger's long bones, concentrating on the thighs and forearms.

'Oh,' she says, looking at the screen, 'your baby is waving.'

I sit up but instead of enjoying the moment, I am immediately anxious. 'What are the fingers like? Are they short? Can you scan the hand? You didn't manage to do it last time. Can you check?'

'The hand looks fine,' she says. 'All the fingers are there and the length isn't bad either. The baby's making a fist. Babies with skeletal dysplasia can't make fists, their fingers are too short. So it's looking OK.'

She carries on for another five minutes, moving the probe silently over my tummy, while I lie there and slowly digest the information. She examined the head and the chest last time I was here and said that they looked all right, and now the hands are looking good.

Dr Chitty finishes up and tells me to wait next door. Five minutes later she arrives to deliver her verdict.

'Well,' she says, 'your baby seems to be growing. It is still small, the long bones are still short, particularly the femur and ulna, but I don't think it looks like it has skeletal dysplasia.'

'You don't?'

'Not in a severe form anyway.'

'Right,' I say. For some reason I am now crying. I can feel tears rolling down my cheeks. But I carry on talking. 'So things are OK?'

'Put it this way, I am not too worried,' she says. 'And I am going to cancel your appointment at Great Ormond Street. You will still need to have your baby checked out when it's born,' she continues, 'and you will still need to keep an eye on it. It still may have some problems. But as far as I can tell, it's just a small baby.'

'A bit of a short-arse,' I suggest, 'who might need to turn its trousers up?'

'Something like that.' She smiles.

I leave the hospital in a fog of emotion. Our baby could be fine, after all. I can't believe it. I'm shocked and exhausted and not really able to deal with the information. I call Less Attractive to share the possibly good news.

'Now look what you've done,' he says. His voice is very quiet indeed. 'I'm in a very important meeting and you've made me cry.'

33

I have a week to go and I'm really beginning to feel it. Despite the fact that I am having a small baby and am not that large, I feel absolutely enormous. Sitting is impossible, lying down is unbearable and moving is exhausting. My back hurts, my knees are sore and my ankles are so fat and puffy I've got legs like pig's trotters. My ability to converse is limited and my sense of humour has long since taken a holiday. It really is time to get this baby out.

I go to visit my extremely charming consultant Mr Teoh at St Mary's Paddington to discuss my birth plan. The only problem is I don't have one. He runs through my options and sits expectantly rubbing his hands, while I stare vacantly back at him. I know some women have the whole thing totally sorted, from the music they want to the nightie they'll wear and the rubber ball they'll give birth on. I, on the other hand, have only just managed to wash my pyjamas.

'So,' says Mr Teoh again. 'What's the plan?'

'I want a natural birth,' I hear myself saying. 'But I don't want to wait long after my due date so I would like to be induced.'

'OK.' He nods. 'I'll book you in for . . .' He pauses and looks through his papers. 'How does Monday evening sound for you?'

'Monday evening sounds fine,' I confirm, as if I am ordering a new bathroom suite or a takeaway pizza. I even check my diary, like I might be busy that day. 'That sounds good.'

'OK.' He smiles again. 'See you then.'

I wander out of his office and call up Less Attractive, telling him that it's all go for Monday and that I've booked an induction.

'Why have you done that?' he queries.

'I have absolutely no idea,' I reply.

'I think you are going mad,' he suggests.

'I think you might be right,' I reply.

The next day the full implications of what I have done suddenly dawn on me. What was I thinking, booking an induction? As if I haven't had enough interference as it is. What's the hurry? Apart from being fed up with the whole thing, what was my motivation? Most of my girlfriends are a little shocked when I tell them.

'Why have you done that?' they all ask.

'I have absolutely no idea,' I reply. 'I don't think I was concentrating and it seemed like a good thing to say at the time. It made me sound like I had some sort of plan, no matter how poorly thought through it was.'

With the threat of induction looming and all the drugs that entails, I have become determined to see if the Passenger can be coaxed into the world by more user-friendly methods. The first thing I do is go to see a cranial osteopath called Fabi in his practice just off Regent's Park. He is charming and delightful and with the gentle laying-on of hands that appears to do nothing he immediately cures my chronic backache and hopefully gets the whole birth process a bit more on track.

The next day I return to my wonderful acupuncturist, who has been treating me right from the very barren beginning. It seems only proper and, actually, rather amazing that Justine is also there at the end. It is lovely to see her, and as well as putting needles in interesting places to get things moving she gives me some tips on the birth. She suggests arnica tablets for post birth, some lavender oil on a cold flannel during it and raspberry leaf tea to get the show on the road. She also suggests the inevitable – curry and sex.

Less Attractive's shoulders sink when I relay this. In fact, judging by the lemon-sucking look on his face, it's like I have asked him to bed a whale, which in a way I suppose I have. To say he is not keen has to be the understatement of the year. The first night he finds an excuse to go out and doesn't return until way past midnight. The second, I slightly let him off the hook. I order a chicken tikka massala as my induction curry and he declares that a massala is not going to get anything moving, least of all a baby, so the whole sex thing is clearly pointless. I try to protest but I don't really have a leg to stand on. Perhaps if I had gone for the vindaloo he might have been turned on by my determination, but the sissy curry was clearly not cutting it.

So now it's all down to me. I'm drinking raspberry tea by the gallon and bathing in an essential oil, clary sage. I have reflexology booked for this afternoon. But I don't hold out much hope. As if someone tweaking my feet is going to shift this little Passenger. But at this stage in the proceedings I'm prepared to try anything, except a stinking hot Madras.

34

I never made it to the reflexology. A couple of hours before my appointment the contractions started. They were quite mild at first, like a pang of chronic wind that shot right through me and then disappeared as quickly as it came. They were so weak and dull that I managed to watch a whole Friday night's television, snack on taramasalata and crisps and go to bed.

By 6am, however, things were really beginning to move. The pain was a whole lot worse, shooting right through my body in sharp waves causing my head to momentarily blow off, but the contractions were still about fifteen minutes apart. As

I sat down in the chair, gripping the arms, I remember thinking this was going to be a long, long day.

Less Attractive and I did not know what to do. Whether to try actually to achieve something, go for a walk, go out for lunch, decorate the nursery. Or whether simply to stay in, stare at the wall and wait for things to get worse. Fortunately we chose the wall option. By midday I was shrieking like some nutter in a primitive torture chamber. Every time I was gripped by a wave of pain I would rise out of my chair and attempt to surf it, like some uncoordinated boogie boarder who had eaten all the pies. The moments in between were spent slumped forward catching my breath as Less Attractive chatted away with hysterical good humour, filling the hours with banter. There was something on the television but, rather like a football match, it didn't make any impression on me.

Come 3pm Less Attractive snapped and called the hospital. He was tentatively insistent but they refused to consider my coming in until my contractions were no more than five minutes apart; mine had a rhythm of their own but they certainly weren't that regular.

Three hours later and I could not bear it any more. Having rather blithely informed anyone who was still talking to me in the run-up to the birth that I rather liked pain (I'd had a couple of tattoos in my youth, for chrissake) and that I was looking forward to it, I now realized I had been talking a total load of breathtakingly stupid bollocks. I don't like pain at all. Pain is miserable. Pain is sore. Pain bloody hurts. And no amount of popping Nurofen or biting on a leather strap (don't ask – if it was good enough for John Wayne . . .) was making a blind bit of difference. I needed to get to hospital right now!

Less Attractive drove like a bat out of hell to St Mary's while I writhed away on the front seat like a walrus. He dumped me outside the hospital and left me clinging on to a lamppost while he parked the car, and then practically dragged me up the steps to the maternity unit. I was in so much pain I was clearly about to give birth then and there in the bare blue-painted corridor. They whisked me to a bed in a small sort of holding bay, next to another couple who were about to pop, and gave me an examination. I was one centimetre dilated.

'What?' I screeched, purple in the face. 'One? One? Are you sure it's just one?'

The nurse nodded.

'All that work and screaming and agony and I am only one bloody centimetre dilated. You mean I've got another nine to go?' I looked as pink and puffed and incredulous as I sounded. 'I don't bloody believe it.' I slumped back on the bed, furious.

'When did your waters break?' asked the nurse.

'They haven't,' I barked.

'They have,' she replied.

'Oh,' I said. 'I thought I'd just become incontinent.'

'No,' she replied. 'I need someone to check you again.'

'Great . . .' I inhaled. I couldn't finish the pissed-off end of my sentence before having to start panting.

When I was examined again it transpired that my cervix had got stuck, and with a bit of tweaking it suddenly sprang out another two centimetres. However, the Passenger was in some distress and had released muconium into my waters, which meant that they needed to get the baby out relatively quickly.

Left once more to moan and writhe on the bed, I screamed to Less Attractive that I needed some gas and air. He fumbled around behind me looking for tubes. Eventually he handed me something that reminded me of going scuba-diving and I inhaled into the contraction. It did nothing. I inhaled again. Still nothing. I inhaled, exhaled, inhaled, exhaled sounding like Darth Vader, and still nothing except a large wave of nausea. This gas stuff was rubbish. I needed to get some *proper bloody pain relief right bloody now.*

Eventually I was taken to a private room and someone shoved a great fat needle in my spine. The relief was extraordinary. The cavewoman who had been moaning and flailing around the room, growling in pain, was put back in her box and my normal fairly pleasant personality re-emerged. I lay back in my bed, was introduced to my midwife Theodora, and was hooked up to a whole load of machines. We were then left to get on with it.

The rest of the night was a bit of a blur. I remember being full of drugs, watching the clock opposite seemingly leap forward hours at a time. I remember talking to Theodora about Zimbabwean politics, as everyone does when they're in labour. I remember sending Less Attractive home because I had run out of things to talk to him about. But what I remember most of all is my baby's heartbeat. Wired up to a monitor because of the epidural and other drugs to get the contractions going, I felt like the Passenger was already here. In the early hours of the morning, as I lay there shivering, my teeth chattering, it was the most comforting sound I have ever heard. I can still hear it now, months later, when I close my eyes and concentrate. The little determined beats, belting away. It was like the baby was knocking on the door of life, asking to come in. I shall never forget it.

At six thirty I was told that I was ten centimetres dilated and should start to push. Less Attractive, fresh from two hours' sleep, took up position, got out his trusty lavender flannel and began to mop my brow. I pushed and pushed and was getting nowhere. I pushed again and still nothing. I then decided to embrace my inner cave bitch whom I had banished earlier and, despite the fact that my body was dead from the waist down, I hauled myself up on to all fours. I strained and pushed and yelled at Less Attractive. I told him to 'Fuck off with his damp lavender fucking flannel on my forehead' and 'All I need now is a frizzy fucking fringe.' And still there was nothing. Then Theodora ignited the fuse.

'Your baby is tired,' she said. 'If you don't push it out soon, you will have to have a Caesarean.'

That was it. I have never pushed so hard in my life. My face went bright red. I thought my eyeballs were going to pop out over the bedhead I strained so much. And then five minutes later this squirming, thrusting, pushing little slithery grey thing landed on my tummy. It was so forceful as it pushed its way up my stomach, so very keen to be here. I was overwhelmed.

'It's a girl,' said Theodora.

'What?' I said. 'But I'm having a boy.'

'It's a girl,' grinned Less Attractive, silently uncrossing his fingers.

'I don't understand?' I said. Leaning forward, I picked her up by the waist and tipped her upside down. She was indeed a girl. 'Hello,' I smiled, kissing her very wet, very grey, very crumpled little face. 'I am so happy to meet you. We've been waiting for you for a very long time.'

Less Attractive burst into tears while I'm afraid I was so stunned I didn't really know what to do. I just lay there squeezing my little girl so tightly, not wanting to let her go. She smelt so delicious, she felt so soft and warm and wonderful. I couldn't really believe it. All this time, all this waiting, all this agony, all the injections, the drugs, the change of blood and the worry, the tears, the pain and here she was, her little grey hands clinging on to my chest. It was all worth it.

'She's OK,' said Less Attractive.

'What?' I mumbled.

'The doctors say she's fine,' he said.

'Not short?'

'Not short.' He smiled.

'Not small?'

'She's not huge. She's six pounds four ounces. But she's all right.'

A few minutes later, she was taken away to be cleaned up and then returned to Less Attractive all wrapped up in a blue blanket. I remember he looked as if he were going to burst with pride as he very gently kissed her soft, fragile head.

'You did it!' He grinned, showing me her pink, wrinkled, swaddled little face. 'Look at her. She's perfect. We're a family.' He smiled. 'At last.'

There is such a thing as a happy ending. Even when you're just at the beginning . . .

Epilogue

Six months on and it is hard to imagine life without Allegra Carmen Elizabeth Allen. She is a feisty little ball of fun with large brown eyes, tufts of dark curls and the sort of long dark lashes that Liza Minnelli would be proud of. She is still quite small but she is delightfully noisy. Her trills and coos fill our house on a daily basis. She is fond of carrot, but not overly keen on peas, and appears to be chubbing up nicely. She is also, obviously, extremely clever and talented. She can blow a raspberry with her tongue, roll one way and is a whiz with her rattle. Even her rapidly accumulating pile of multicoloured plastic tat only serves to make our bourgeois minimalist semi a whole lot more interesting.

In the end, we did get asked to attend the Genetics Unit at Great Ormond Street Hospital. There, we met six of the UK's finest and kindest doctors. They weighed Allegra, measured her, undressed her and played with her and said what Less Attractive and I had hoped all along – that she was perfect. In fact, she has confounded us all. They said they didn't know why she looked so small on her scans. They said that there was no real explanation for it, that sometimes these things just happen. They told us they didn't want to see us again and all Less Attractive and I could do was smile. Never has a dismissal been greeted with such joy. Then again, never has an arrival either.